Department of Veterans Affairs
Health Services Research & Development Service

Evidence-based Synthesis Program

Advanced Wound Care Therapies for Non-Healing Diabetic, Venous, and Arterial Ulcers: A Systematic Review

November 2012

Prepared for:
Department of Veterans Affairs
Veterans Health Administration
Quality Enhancement Research Initiative
Health Services Research & Development Service
Washington, DC 20420

Prepared by:
Evidence-based Synthesis Program (ESP) Center
Minneapolis VA Medical Center
Minneapolis, MN
Timothy J. Wilt, M.D., M.P.H., Director

Investigators:
Principal Investigators:
Nancy Greer, Ph.D.
Neal Foman, M.D., M.S.
Timothy Wilt, M.D., M.P.H.

Co-Investigators:
James Dorrian, B.S.
Patrick Fitzgerald, M.P.H.
Roderick MacDonald, M.S.

Research Assistant:
Indy Rutks, B.S.

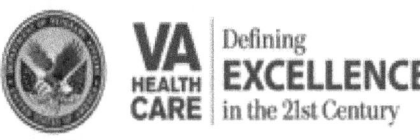

PREFACE

Quality Enhancement Research Initiative's (QUERI) Evidence-based Synthesis Program (ESP) was established to provide timely and accurate syntheses of targeted healthcare topics of particular importance to Veterans Affairs (VA) managers and policymakers, as they work to improve the health and healthcare of Veterans. The ESP disseminates these reports throughout VA.

QUERI provides funding for four ESP Centers and each Center has an active VA affiliation. The ESP Centers generate evidence syntheses on important clinical practice topics, and these reports help:

- develop clinical policies informed by evidence,
- guide the implementation of effective services to improve patient outcomes and to support VA clinical practice guidelines and performance measures, and
- set the direction for future research to address gaps in clinical knowledge.

In 2009, the ESP Coordinating Center was created to expand the capacity of QUERI Central Office and the four ESP sites by developing and maintaining program processes. In addition, the Center established a Steering Committee comprised of QUERI field-based investigators, VA Patient Care Services, Office of Quality and Performance, and Veterans Integrated Service Networks (VISN) Clinical Management Officers. The Steering Committee provides program oversight, guides strategic planning, coordinates dissemination activities, and develops collaborations with VA leadership to identify new ESP topics of importance to Veterans and the VA healthcare system.

Comments on this evidence report are welcome and can be sent to Nicole Floyd, ESP Coordinating Center Program Manager, at nicole.floyd@va.gov.

Recommended citation: Greer N, Foman N, Dorrian J, Fitzgerald P, MacDonald R, Rutks I, Wilt T. Advanced Wound Care Therapies for Non-Healing Diabetic, Venous, and Arterial Ulcers: A Systematic Review. VA-ESP Project #09-009; 2012.

TABLE OF CONTENTS

EXECUTIVE SUMMARY

BACKGROUND

Chronic ulcers (i.e., ulcers that are unresponsive to initial therapy or that persist despite appropriate care) are estimated to affect over 6 million people in the United States. The incidence is expected to increase as the population ages and as the number of individuals with diabetes increases. Chronic ulcers negatively affect the quality of life and productivity of the patient and represent a substantial financial burden to the health care system.

Lower extremity ulcers, especially those attributed to either diabetes, venous disease, or arterial disease comprise a substantial proportion of chronic ulcers. Approximately 15% to 25% of individuals with diabetes develop a foot ulcer at some point in their lifetime and an estimated 12% of those patients require lower extremity amputation. Healing is complicated by diabetic neuropathy and susceptibility to infection. Venous disease accounts for the majority of chronic lower extremity ulcers. Venous hypertension secondary to various cuases results in damage to vessel walls and ultimately leads to skin breakdown. Arterial ulcers are less common and are a result of impaired circulation which can affect healing lead to ulceration.

Standard treatment for diabetic ulcers includes debridement of necrotic tissue, infection control, local ulcer care, mechanical off-loading, management of blood glucose levels, and education on foot care. For venous ulcers, standard treatment typically includes the use of mechanical compression and limb elevation to reverse tissue edema and improve venous blood flow. Care for ulcers caused by arterial insufficiency is centered on reestablishing blood flow and minimizing further loss of tissue perfusion.

If ulcers do not adequately heal with standard treatment, additional modalities may be required – these are often termed "advanced wound care therapies." Lower extremity ulcers are frequently classified etiologically as diabetic, venous or arterial, though overlap may exist. Treatment modalities and wound care therapies are often selected based on the ulcer characteristics as well as patient factors, past treatment, and provider preference. A large and growing array of advanced wound care therapies of different composition and indications have been developed though their efficacy, comparative effectiveness and harm is not well established.

The purpose of this review is to synthesize the evidence on therapies for non-healing diabetic, venous, and arterial lower extremity ulcers. This work was nominated by Rajiv Jain, MD (Chief Consultant, Office of Patient Care Services) and Jeffrey Robbins, DPM (Director, Podiatry Service) and is intended to provide an evidence base to guide clinical practice and policy needs within the VA. We recognize that a non-healing ulcer is likely a result of multiple factors and comorbid conditions. We group studies in the review according to the study authors' description of the included ulcer type. The review focuses on FDA-approved therapies and examines clinically relevant outcomes. We address the following key questions:

Key Question #1. What are the efficacy and harms of therapies for diabetic ulcers? Is efficacy dependent on ancillary therapies? Does efficacy differ according to patient demographics, comorbid conditions, treatment compliance, or activity level?

1

Key Question #2. What are the efficacy and harms of therapies for venous ulcers? Is efficacy dependent on ancillary therapies? Does efficacy differ according to patient demographics, comorbid conditions, treatment compliance, or activity level?

Key Question #3. What are the efficacy and harms of therapies for arterial ulcers? Is efficacy dependent on ancillary therapies? Does efficacy differ according to patient demographics, comorbid conditions, treatment compliance, or activity level?

Advanced wound care therapies included in this review are: collagen, biological dressings, biological skin equivalents, keratinocytes, platelet-derived growth factor, platelet-rich plasma, silver products, intermittent pneumatic compression therapy, negative pressure wound therapy, electromagnetic therapy, hyperbaric oxygen, topical oxygen, and ozone oxygen. We included studies that compared these therapies to standard care (as defined above) as well as to other advanced therapies. We recognize that collagen may be used as a vehicle for the delivery of other therapies (e.g., growth factors, silver). Under the collagen heading, we report findings from studies of collagen used as an inert matrix material.

METHODS

We searched MEDLINE (OVID) for randomized controlled trials (RCTs) published from 1995 through August, 2012 using standard search terms. We limited the search to studies involving human subjects over age 18 and published in the English language. Search terms included skin ulcer, foot ulcer, leg ulcer, varicose ulcer, diabetic ulcer, diabetic foot, wound healing, venous insufficiency, artificial skin, biological dressings, negative-pressure wound therapy, collagen, silver, topical oxygen, hyperbaric oxygen, electromagnetic, platelet-derived growth factor, platelet-rich plasma, and intermittent pneumatic compression devices. Investigators and research associates trained in the critical analysis of literature assessed for relevance the abstracts of citations identified from literature searches. We obtained additional articles from a search of the Cochrane Library, existing systematic reviews, and reference lists of pertinent studies.

Study, patient, ulcer and treatment characteristics, primary and secondary outcomes, and adverse events were extracted by trained research associates under the supervision of the Principal Investigator. Our primary outcome was the percentage of ulcers healed at study completion. Additional "primary outcomes" included time to complete ulcer healing, patient global assessment, and return to daily activities. Secondary outcomes included ulcer infection, amputation, revascularization surgery, ulcer recurrence, time to ulcer recurrence, pain or discomfort, hospitalization, progression to require home care, quality of life, all-cause mortality, adverse events, and adverse reactions to treatment. Where feasible, pooled analyses were performed for outcomes from studies of equivalent therapies used to treat like ulcer types. We calculated absolute risk differences for the primary outcome of ulcers healed. All other data were narratively summarized. We assessed quality of individual studies according to established criteria for randomized controlled trials. Strength of evidence was determined for primary outcomes.

DATA SYNTHESIS

We constructed evidence tables showing study, patient, and intervention characteristics; methodological quality; and outcomes, organized by ulcer type (diabetic, venous, arterial) and then by treatment. We analyzed studies to compare their characteristics, methods, and findings. We compiled a summary of findings for each ulcer type based on qualitative and semi-quantitative synthesis of the findings. We identified and highlighted findings from VA or Department of Defense (DoD) populations.

PEER REVIEW

A draft version of this report was reviewed by clinical content experts, as well as clinical leadership. Reviewer comments were addressed and our responses are incorporated in the final report.

RESULTS

We screened 1,230 titles and abstracts, excluded 1,053, and performed a more detailed review on 177 articles. From these, we identified 68 articles representing 64 randomized controlled trials (RCTs) (35 trials involved patients with diabetic ulcers, 20 with venous ulcers, 1 with arterial ulcers, and 8 with mixed etiology or amputation ulcers) that addressed one of the key questions. Most studies compared advanced wound care therapies to standard care or placebo. Direct comparison of one advanced wound care therapy to another was done in 10 of 35 studies (29%) of diabetic ulcers, 4 of 20 studies (20%) of venous ulcers, and 2 of 9 studies (22%) of arterial or mixed ulcers. Overall, studies enrolled a diverse group of participants as determined by age, gender and race/ethnicity. The majority of enrollees were male, white, aged 60 years and older, and demographics did not differ markedly by ulcer type. However, studies rarely reported results separately by important baseline characteristics.

In studies of diabetic ulcers, mean ulcer sizes ranged from 1.9 to 41.5 cm^2, however, the mean ulcer size was greater than 10 cm^2 in only 6 of 29 studies reporting ulcer size. Mean ulcer durations ranged from 14.5 days to 21.6 months with durations of greater than 1 year in 6 of 21 studies reporting. In studies of venous ulcers, mean ulcer sizes ranged from 1.2 to 11.1 cm^2 in 16 studies reporting with 4 of 16 studies reporting mean ulcer sizes of greater than 10 cm^2. Ulcer durations ranged from 7 weeks to 626 weeks with durations of greater than 1 year in 6 of 11 studies reporting ulcer duration. The mean ulcer size in the single study of arterial ulcers was 4.8 cm^2; ulcer duration was not reported. In the single amputation wound study, the mean ulcer size was 20.7 cm^2 with of a mean duration of 1.5 months.

Key Question #1. What are the efficacy and harms of therapies for diabetic ulcers? Is efficacy dependent on ancillary therapies? Does efficacy differ according to patient demographics, comorbid conditions, treatment compliance, or activity level?

We identified 35 eligible trials of 9 different advanced wound care therapies for diabetic ulcers. In 26 of these trials the ulcer was described as a "foot" ulcer, in 7 trials the ulcer was described as a "lower extremity" ulcer, and in 2 trials the ulcer was described only as a "diabetic ulcer." The ulcer type was further described as neuropathic in 11 trials, ischemic in 1 trial, neuroischemic in 1 trial, and mixed in 3 trials. Of the remaining trials, 16 had inclusion criteria related to adequate circulation or exclusion criteria related to severe arterial disease and 3 did not specify criteria related to circulation.

Collagen (4 RCTs)

Four RCTs (n=489 randomized) reported outcomes of interest. All were rated as fair quality. One study (n=86) found collagen (Graftjacket) to significantly improve ulcer healing compared to standard care (70% healed in the biological dressing group, 46% in the standard care group; ARD=23%, 95% CI 3% to 44%). This difference was maintained after adjusting for baseline ulcer size. Three trials found no significant difference between collagen matrix products and standard care in the percentage of ulcers healed (differences of 9% to 14% between groups). No study found collagen to improve time to complete ulcer healing at study completion (3 studies reporting, differences of 0.4, 1.1, and 1.2 weeks). Two studies reported no significant difference between collagen treatment and standard care for ulcers infected during treatment. No differences were observed in withdrawals due to adverse events (3 studies, 7% overall, 6% versus 0%, and 6% versus 5%) or all-cause mortality (two studies, 1.4% versus 4.3% and 0% overall). One study reported no difference between groups in amputation or need for revascularization surgery.

Biological Dressings (2 RCTs)

Two studies (n=124 randomized), both multisite RCTs, were identified. Both studies, one of which was a non-inferiority study, showed no difference between a biological dressing and other advanced wound care therapies. Neither study found a difference in mean time to healing and no statistical differences were seen between biological dressings and PDGF in the type or number of adverse events. Only one study reported on the possible effect of patient characteristics on efficacy. Results from an *a priori* subgroup analysis indicated that the biological dressing did not improve healing (p=0.14) of plantar surface ulcers more than the advanced therapy comparator (PDGF). A second subgroup analysis found that biological dressing significantly healed more ulcers in patients with type 2 (p=0.03) but not type 1 diabetes.

Biological Skin Equivalents (7 RCTs)

In three fair quality studies (n=576 randomized), Dermagraft statistically significantly improved ulcer healing compared to standard care in two of the trials (30% versus 18% in one study, 50% versus 8% in the other), one of which also reported a significant faster time to closure. The third trial found significant differences in ulcer healing only in patients receiving metabolically active Dermagraft. In this older trial, some Dermagraft samples had a level of metabolic activity outside of the therapeutic range. All of the trials allowed for up to 8 pieces of Dermagraft. A pooled analysis showed an overall non-significant benefit of Dermagraft compared to standard care for ulcer healing (RR=1.49, 95% CI 0.96 to 2.32, I^2=43%). A fourth study, a small trial (n=26) of poor quality, allowed for up to 3 grafts and found no difference in ulcer healing between Dermagraft and a biological dressing. Two fair quality studies (n=359 randomized) compared Apligraf to standard care and showed significant benefits in ulcer healing (55% versus 34%; ARD=21%, 95% CI 9% to 32%; RR=1.58, 95% CI 1.20 to 2.08, I^2=0%). One trial allowed up to 5 treatments over 5 weeks while the other allowed up to 3 treatments over 8 weeks. A small (n=29 ulcers), poor-quality study compared up to 5 Apligraf treatments to cryopreserved split-thickness skin allograft and showed patients benefited from both therapies, although a larger percentage of ulcers healed with the allograft. No statistical analyses were provided. Two of the Dermagraft studies reported on factors associated with ulcer healing. In one study, neither patient age, gender, ulcer size or duration, diabetes type, ankle-arm index, nor HbA_1c were significantly associated with time to closure. In another study, an interim analysis showed a relationship between ulcer duration and healing and therefore the analysis focused on ulcers of greater than 6 weeks duration. This study also reported outcomes based on ulcer location. Although both analyses resulted in non-significant differences, there was a trend for more forefoot/toe ulcers (n=214) to heal with Dermagraft (29.5% versus 19.6%, p=0.065). For heel ulcers (n=31), 33% of those treated with Dermagraft achieved closure compared to 8% in the control group (p=0.01). Four studies found no difference in recurrence between either Dermagraft or Apligraf and standard care. One study reported fewer amputations in the Apligraf group compared to standard care; a second study reported no difference. Overall, the number of adverse events was low with no differences between treatment groups.

Platelet-Derived Wound Healing (Platelet-Derived Growth Factors [PDGF]) (9 RCTs)

Nine RCTs (n=990 randomized) compared PDGF to placebo gel or standard ulcer care (n=6), an advanced wound care therapy (n=2), or both (n=1). Two studies were of poor quality, five were of fair quality, and two were of good quality. Compared to standard care (7 trials), PDGF demonstrated a greater percentage of healed ulcers at study completion, although there was evidence of substantial heterogeneity (58% versus 37%; ARD=21%, 95% CI 14% to 29%; RR=1.45, 95% CI 1.03 to 2.05, I^2=85%). In five studies reporting, time to ulcer healing was significantly shorter in the PDGF treated groups in four studies (29 to 41 days; p≤0.01) with one study reporting no difference. However, when compared to silver sulfadiazine, sodium carboxymethylcellulose gel, or biological dressing there was no significant difference in percentage of ulcers healed or time to healing. Several studies looked at factors associated with ulcer healing. In one study, ulcers less than 9 cm^2, ulcers located on non-weight-bearing surfaces, and the use of antibiotics significantly improved healing. Another study reported that healing did not vary by age and baseline HbA_1c but that compliance with off-loading was positively associated with healing (p not reported). No studies reported significant differences between treatment arms for secondary outcomes or adverse events.

Platelet-Rich Plasma (PRP) (2 RCTs)

One poor quality and one fair quality study (n=96 randomized) evaluated the efficacy of PRP compared to placebo or another advance wound therapy (platelet poor plasma, PPP). PRP was applied twice per week for up to 12 weeks in one study and up to 20 weeks in the other study. Neither study demonstrated a significant effect on the percentage of ulcers healed (PRP compared to placebo: 33% versus 28% healed; PRP compared to PPP: 100% versus 75% healed). One study reported a significantly shorter time to healed ulcers for PRP compared to PPP (11.5 weeks versus 17.0 weeks, p<0.005) and the other showed no significant difference between PRP and placebo (43 days versus 47 days). One study reported on secondary outcomes of interest and adverse events with no difference between PRP and placebo.

Silver Products (4 RCTs)

We identified four fair quality RCTs (n=280 randomized) of silver products; three were versus another advanced wound care product. Three studies reported healed ulcers with mixed results. In one study (n=66), ulcers treated with silver ointment were more likely to heal than those treated with standard care (39% versus 16%; ARD=23%, 95% CI 2% to 43%); in the other 2 studies, there was no difference in healing between silver products (dressing or cream) versus oak bark extract or a calcium-based dressing. There were no differences between silver dressing and calcium dressing or silver cream and poly-herbal cream for time to ulcer healing. No differences between silver dressing or creams and either standard care or other advanced wound care therapies were observed for our secondary outcomes and adverse events of interest.

Negative Pressure Wound Therapy (NPWT) (3 RCTs)

Three RCTs (n=418 randomized) compared NPWT to standard care. One study was of good quality, one appeared to be of moderate quality but reporting was limited, one was a small pilot study. Only the good quality study (n=335 with primary outcome) reported on the percentage of healed ulcers finding improved healing in the NPWT group compared to standard care of advanced moist wound therapy (43% versus 29%; ARD=14%, 95% CI 4% to 24%). All three studies reported on the time to healing and found mixed results. In the good quality study, NPWT reduced second amputations compared to advanced moist wound therapy (4.1% versus 10.2%, p=0.04). The moderate quality study reported a significant positive effect of NPWT on mental and physical health compared to standard care. No differences in adverse events were observed in any study although reporting was sparse.

Hyperbaric Oxygen Therapy (HBOT) (5 RCTs)

Five RCTs of fair quality, enrolling a total of 326 subjects, met inclusion criteria. Four studies (n=240) compared HBOT to standard or sham therapy. The findings could not be pooled due to variations in follow-up duration. Three studies with at least one year of follow-up reported a significantly higher percentage of ulcers healed (using Fisher's exact test) among patients allocated to adjunctive HBOT (range 52% to 66%) than sham therapy or standard care (range 0% to 29%). In one of the studies, all of the standard therapy patients required some form of surgical management (i.e., debridement, graft or flap, or distal amputation) to achieve ulcer closure compared to 16% of patients in the HBOT group. A short-term trial found that, within 2 weeks of therapy, 2 of 14 patients had complete healing versus none of the 13 patients in the standard care control group; the difference was not significant. None of the studies reported mean time to healing. Two studies reported no difference in amputations required between HBOT and sham therapy; one study reported fewer amputations in the HBOT group compared to the standard therapy group. Adverse events were similar between the HBOT and standard care/sham groups. HBOT resulted in significantly less healing (25% versus 55%, p=0.008) than extracorporeal shock wave therapy (EST) in one poor quality study.

Ozone-Oxygen Therapy (1 RCT)

One RCT of fair quality (n=61 randomized) compared ozone-oxygen therapy to sham treatments and found no significant difference between groups in the proportion of patients with completely healed ulcers (41% versus 34%, p=0.34). Post-hoc subgroup findings in patients with ulcers of 5 cm² or less found that active treatment resulted in 100% closure compared to 50% in the sham treatment group (p=0.006). No differences were reported between active and sham therapy for ulcers infected during treatment, amputation, or withdrawals due to adverse events.

Summary

Nine different advanced wound care therapies used for treatment of diabetic ulcers provided information on our primary and secondary outcomes. Most compared outcomes to standard care, placebo or sham treatments with few reporting comparative effectiveness findings versus other advanced wound care therapies. Advanced wound care therapies included collagen, biological dressings, biological skin equivalents, platelet-derived growth factors, platelet-rich plasma, silver products, negative pressure wound therapy, hyperbaric oxygen therapy, and ozone-oxygen therapy. We summarize our primary and secondary outcome findings below. We found insufficient evidence to address the question whether efficacy and comparative effectiveness differed according to patient demographics, comorbid conditions, treatment compliance, or activity level.

Primary Outcomes

Advanced wound care therapies using platelet-rich plasma or ozone oxygen therapy did not improve diabetic ulcer healing compared to standard care (2 studies) or another advanced care therapy (1 study). Other therapies provided mixed results. Four studies compared collagen products to standard care with only one study reporting significantly better healing in the collagen group (70% versus 46%, p=0.03). Pooled results from three studies indicate that the biological skin equivalent Dermagraft compared to standard care results in a non-significant improvement in ulcer healing favoring Dermagraft (35% versus 24%, low strength of evidence, see Executive Summary Table 1). We found moderate strength of evidence that the biological skin equivalent, bi-layer Apligraf, improved healing compared to standard care (55% versus 34%, p=0.001; 2 studies). While pooled results from studies of platelet-derived growth factor showed improvement in the percentage of ulcers healed compared to placebo or standard care (58% versus 37%, p=0.04; 7 studies) the strength of evidence was low due to high heterogeneity of results between studies. One good quality study provided moderate strength evidence that negative pressure wound therapy improved healing more than standard care (43% versus 29%, p<0.05). Three long-term, fair quality studies of HBOT reported significantly better healing with HBOT (52% to 66%) than sham therapy or standard care (0% to 29%).

Few studies reported time to ulcer healing and other primary outcomes. We found no benefit in time to ulcer healing for collagen, biological dressings, or silver products. We found mixed but generally negative results for biological skin equivalents (1 of 4 Dermagraft and 1 of 3 Apligraf studies showing benefit compared to standard care), platelet-derived growth factors (4 of 8 studies reporting showing benefit compared to placebo or standard care), platelet-rich plasma (1 of 2 studies showing benefit compared to another advanced therapy), and negative pressure wound therapy (1 of 3 studies showing benefit compared to standard care). Strength of evidence was low or insufficient for all findings related to time to ulcer healing. One study of a silver dressing versus a calcium dressing reported a global outcome of healed or improved ulcers with no difference between groups. No studies reported on return to daily activities.

Secondary Outcomes

The most commonly reported secondary outcomes were ulcers infected during treatment and ulcer recurrence. No study reported a benefit for these outcomes for any of the advanced therapies reviewed. Fewer amputations were reported in three studies (one each of a biological skin equivalent, negative pressure wound therapy, and hyperbaric oxygen therapy all compared to standard care) while five studies reported no difference. Few studies reported other secondary outcomes of interest including revascularization or surgery, pain or discomfort, hospitalization, need for home care, or quality of life. No significant differences between treatment groups (including 12 studies comparing an advanced therapy to standard care, 3 studies comparing one advanced therapy to another advanced therapy, and 1 study with both standard therapy and advanced therapy comparison arms) were seen in all-cause mortality though studies were not designed to assess this outcome. We found no significant differences in study withdrawals due to adverse events or allergic reactions to treatment.

Advanced Wound Care Therapies for Non-Healing Diabetic, Venous, and Arterial Ulcers: A Systematic Review

Executive Summary Table 1. Strength of Evidence – Advanced Wound Care Therapies for Diabetic Ulcers

Treatment	Control(s)	Outcome	Number of Studies (n for Primary Outcome)*	Comments	Strength of Evidence
Collagen	Standard care	Percentage of ulcers healed	4 (483)	One study reported significant improvement compared to standard care. Three studies reported no significant difference between collagen and standard care. Trials were rated as fair quality.	Low
		Mean time to ulcer healing		One trial found a significant difference favoring standard care; two found no difference.	Low
Biological Dressings	Advanced therapy control (*PDGF, BSE*)	Percentage of ulcers healed	2 (99)	Two fair quality trials showed no difference compared to other advanced wound care therapies.	Low
		Mean time to ulcer healing		No trial was significantly different versus control.	Low
Biological Skin Equivalents [BSE] – *Dermagraft*	Standard care	Percentage of ulcers healed	3 (505)	A trend toward statistically significant improvement compared to standard care (RR=1.49, 95% CI 0.96 to 2.32, I^2=43%). Trials were rated as fair quality.	Low
		Mean time to ulcer healing		Inconsistent results, with one trial reporting a significant difference versus standard care. Trials were rated as fair quality.	Low
BSE – *Apligraf*	Standard care	Percentage of ulcers healed	2 (279)	Two trials of fair quality found statistically significant improvement versus standard care (RR=1.58, 95% CI 1.20 to 2.08, I^2=0%).	Moderate
		Mean time to ulcer healing		One trial reported a significant difference between *Apligraf* and standard care.	Low
BSE – *Apligraf*	Advanced therapy control (*Skin allografts -Theraskin*)	Percentage of ulcers healed	1 (29 ulcers)	One fair quality trial found no significant difference versus *Theraskin*.	Low
		Mean time to ulcer healing		No significant difference versus *Theraskin*.	Low
Platelet Derived Wound Healing [PDGF]	Placebo /standard care	Percentage of ulcers healed	7 (685)	Overall statistically significant improvement versus placebo (RR 1.45 [95% CI 1.03 to 2.05]) but results were inconsistent (I^2 85%). Overall study quality was rated as fair.	Low
		Mean time to ulcer healing	5 (731)	Overall, PDGF demonstrated shorter duration of time to ulcer healing versus placebo.	Low
PDGF	Advanced therapy control (*BSE, silver, sodium carboxy-methylcellulose*)	Percentage of ulcers healed	3 (189)	No significant differences compared to an advanced therapy comparator. Trials were rated as fair quality.	Low
		Mean time to ulcer healing		No significant differences compared to an advanced therapy comparator.	Low
Platelet-Rich Plasma [PRP]	Placebo gel, Platelet-Poor Plasma	Percentage of ulcers healed	2 (96)	Neither of the studies (fair to poor quality) demonstrated a significant difference between PRP and its respective control.	Low
		Mean time to ulcer healing		Significantly shorter healing time compared to platelet-poor plasma. No significant difference versus placebo gel.	Low

Advanced Wound Care Therapies for Non-Healing Diabetic, Venous, and Arterial Ulcers: A Systematic Review

Treatment	Control(s)	Outcome	Number of Studies (n for Primary Outcome)*	Comments	Strength of Evidence
Silver Products	Standard care or advanced therapy controls (*calcium-based dressing, oak bark extract, polyherbal cream*)	Percentage of ulcers healed	4 (280)	One trial found silver ointment more effective than standard care. Two trials found no difference in healing between a silver cream or dressing and another advanced care product. Studies were of fair quality.	Low
		Mean time to ulcer healing	2 (174)	Two trials found no difference between silver and another advanced wound care product.	Low
Negative Pressure Wound Therapy [NPWT]	Standard care (*Advanced moist wound therapy, saline gauze*)	Percentage of ulcers healed	1 (335)	One trial of good quality found 43% in the NPWT group experienced ulcer healing compared to 29% treated with standard care (RR=1.49, 95% CI 1.11 to 2.01).	Moderate
		Mean time to ulcer healing	3 (432)	Results for time to healing were inconsistent based on 3 trials of mixed quality.	Low
Hyperbaric Oxygen Therapy (HBOT)	Sham or standard care	Percentage of ulcers healed	4 (233)	Three long-term studies of fair quality found significant improvement with adjunctive HBOT versus sham or standard care; one short-term study found no difference.	Low
		Mean time to ulcer healing	-	Outcome not reported.	Insufficient
HBOT	Advanced therapy control (*Extracorporeal shockwave therapy*)	Percentage of ulcers healed	1 (84)	One trial of poor quality found adjunctive HBOT less effective than extracorporeal shockwave therapy.	Low
		Mean time to ulcer healing	-	Outcome not reported.	Insufficient
Ozone-Oxygen Therapy	Sham	Percentage of ulcers healed	1 (61)	One trial of fair quality found no significant difference between ozone-oxygen and sham.	Low
		Mean time to ulcer healing	-	Outcome not reported.	Insufficient

*Number of ulcers evaluated for the primary outcome

The evidence is rated using the following grades: (1) high strength indicates further research is very unlikely to change the confidence in the estimate of effect, meaning that the evidence reflects the true effect; (2) moderate strength denotes further research may change our confidence in the estimate of effect and may change the estimate; (3) low strength indicates further research is very likely to have an important impact on the confidence in the estimate of effect and is likely to change the estimate, meaning there is low confidence that the evidence reflects the true effect; and (4) insufficient, indicating that the evidence is unavailable or does not permit a conclusion.

Key Question #2. What are the efficacy and harms of therapies for venous ulcers? Is efficacy dependent on ancillary therapies? Does efficacy differ according to patient demographics, comorbid conditions, treatment compliance, or activity level?

We identified 20 eligible trials of 9 different advanced wound care therapies for venous ulcers. In 14 trials the ulcer was described as a "leg" ulcer, in 2 trials the ulcer was described as a "lower extremity" ulcer, and 3 trials did not report the ulcer location describing the ulcer only as a "venous ulcer." In 12 trials a diagnosis of venous ulcers was based on clinical signs or symptoms of venous insufficiency. The remaining 8 trials required either patients to have adequate arterial circulation or specifically excluded patients with known arterial insufficiency.

Collagen (1 RCT)

One fair quality small RCT (n=73 randomized) compared collagen to standard care. No significant differences were found between collagen and standard ulcer care for the percentage of ulcers healed by study completion (49% versus 33%, p=0.18; ARD=16%, 95% CI -7% to 38%) though the confidence interval was wide and cannot exclude a clinically meaningful difference. Fewer ulcers were infected during treatment in the collagen group. There were no significant differences between collagen and standard care for pain, the number of withdrawals due to adverse events, or allergic reaction to treatment. The effects of ancillary therapies or patient factors on outcomes were not reported.

Biological Dressings (1 RCT)

We identified one multisite RCT enrolling 120 patients. This fair quality study found that biological dressing, OASIS Wound Matrix, increased complete ulcer healing at 12 weeks compared to standard care (55% versus 34%; ARD=20%, 95% CI 3% to 38%). The benefit of the biological dressing was significantly increased in patients who received ulcer debridement at baseline. At 6 months follow-up, recurrence was significantly less frequent in the biological dressing group than in the standard care group (0% versus 30%, p=0.03). No statistically significant differences were seen in adverse events between groups.

Biological Skin Equivalents (3 RCTs)

We identified three trials, all of fair quality (total n=380) and all comparing a biological skin equivalent to standard care with compression bandage. Two trials evaluated Dermagraft and one evaluated Apligraf. Both studies of Dermagraft were small in size and did not reach statistical significance for our primary efficacy outcomes when compared to standard care including compression bandages. The Apligraf study was a large (n=309), multicenter trial that found significant increases in the proportion of completely healed ulcers (63% versus 49%; ARD=14%, 95% CI 3% to 26%; p=0.02) and reduction in the time to complete healing (61 days versus 181 days, p=0.003) when compared to standard compression bandage therapy. Of the two studies reporting on adverse events, no significant differences were seen between treatment and control groups. One study reported subgroup analyses. In ulcers of more than 6 months duration, Apligraf resulted in faster healing than standard compression bandage therapy (p=0.001). A similar result was observed for patients with ulcers reaching muscle tissue (p=0.003). For both large ulcers (>1000mm^2; p=0.02) and small ulcers (<1000mm^2; p=0.04), Apligraf resulted in faster healing.

Keratinocytes (4 RCTs)

Four RCTs were identified (n=502 randomized). These trials had marked heterogeneity across several important parameters: keratinocyte source (autologous or allogeneic); cellular state of keratinocytes (fresh, frozen, or lysed), comparators (other keratinocyte product, standard of care); and study size, protocols, and quality. One large, fair quality trial demonstrated significant improvements in both proportion of ulcers healed (38% versus 22%, p=0.01) and time to complete healing (176 days versus more than 201 days, p<0.0001) when BioSeed-S (autologous keratinocytes in fibrin sealant) was compared to standard care. In the other studies, no statistical differences in ulcer healing were seen when cryopreserved, cultured epidermal allografts (CEA) were compared with standard compression therapy (fair quality study), cryopreserved CEA were compared to lyophilized CEA (poor quality study), and when lyophilized keratinocytes were compared to standard care in a large, fair quality, multinational study. Pooled results from the two studies with standard care as the comparator yielded a significant benefit of treatment with keratinocytes (38% versus 24%; ARD=14%, 95% CI 5% to 23%; RR=1.57, 95% CI 1.16 to 2.11, I^2=0%). One study reported recurrence with no different between keratinocyte therapy and standard care. Only the two large studies reported adverse events; one demonstrated similar type and frequency of events compared to standard care, and the other reported a total of 9 minor adverse events that were deemed at least "possibly" related to treatment over the 6 month study. In one study, subgroup analyses found the benefit of keratinocytes in achieving ulcer closure was more pronounced in patients with larger ulcers (>10 cm^2) at baseline (25.5% versus 7.7%, p=0.03). Ulcer duration (greater than 12 months versus less than 12 months) did not influence outcomes. A second study found that the likelihood of healing was higher in small ulcers (p<0.001), ulcers decreasing in size between screening and baseline visits (p=0.001), and ulcers in patients with a higher BMI (p=0.02).

Platelet Rich Plasma (PRP) (1 RCT)

One fair quality study (enrolling 86 patients) found no difference between platelet lysate (applied twice per week for up to 9 months) and standard care regarding the percentage of ulcers healed at study completion (79% versus 77%). When the effects of ulcer area, ulcer duration, gender, and ulcer history were analyzed, only ulcer size was a significant factor in time to heal. No other outcomes or harms of interest were reported.

Silver Products (6 RCTs)

Six studies (n=771 randomized) reported on the use of silver products. One good quality study and one fair quality study compared silver cream/ointment to standard care. One fair quality study compared silver cream to copper cream or to placebo copper cream. Overall, no statistically significant difference in ulcer healing was observed with silver therapy (range 21% to 63%) versus standard care or placebo (range 3% to 80%) with evidence of large heterogeneity (RR=1.65, 95% CI 0.54 to 5.03, I^2=84%). Compared to the copper-based cream, the silver-based cream significantly improved healed ulcers (21% versus 0%, p=0.01 with Fisher's exact test). Results were mixed for two studies, both fair quality, that compared a silver dressing to a similar non-silver dressing. One of the trials (n=42) found a higher rate of healing in the silver dressing group compared to the control dressing at 9 weeks (81% versus 48%; ARD=33%, 95%

CI 6% to 61%); a larger trial (n=204) found no difference (60% versus 57%). One study (n=281) comparing two silver dressings also found no difference (17% vs. 15%). Pooled data from two studies of silver versus non-silver dressings show a non-significant outcome and evidence of heterogeneity (RR=1.27, 95% CI 0.80 to 2.01, I^2=67%). Two studies, of fair quality, reported time to ulcer healing when a silver dressing was compared to a non-silver dressing. One found no significant difference; one did not report significance. No differences were observed between silver-based therapies and other treatments or standard care for other outcomes or adverse events. In one study, female gender (p=0.01), and smaller ulcer size (up to 3 cm diameter, p=0.008) were significantly related to ulcer healing. In another study, a significant difference in healing between treatment and control was observed for shallow ulcers (p=0.04) but not for deep ulcers (p=0.29)

Intermittent Pneumatic Compression Therapy (1 RCT)

One fair quality RCT (n=54 randomized) compared intermittent pneumatic compression (IPC) therapy to compression bandaging (Unna's boot). There was no significant difference between IPC and Unna's boot in the percentage of ulcers healed by study completion (71% versus 60%) or pain/discomfort. There were no significant differences between the number of withdrawals due to adverse events or allergic reactions to treatment. An analysis of ulcer healing by ulcer size found that 100% of ulcers less than 3 cm^2 were healed regardless of treatment group.

Electromagnetic Therapy (EMT) (2 RCTs)

Two fair quality trials of EMT versus sham treatment (n=63 randomized) produced mixed results for percentage of ulcers healed. One trial (n=37) reported a significant increase in the percentage of healed ulcers compared to sham after 90 days (67% versus 32%; ARD=35%, 95% CI 5% to 65%). The other trial (n=19) reported no significant difference after 50 days (20% versus 22%). One study also reported lower pain in the EMT group. No other outcomes or adverse events differed between groups.

Hyperbaric Oxygen Therapy (HBOT) (1 RCT)

One small (n=16 randomized) good quality RCT comparing HBOT to sham found no difference between groups. No other outcomes were reported.

Summary

We identified 20 trials of nine different advanced ulcer care therapies for patients with venous ulcers: collagen, biological dressings, biological skin equivalents, keratinocytes, platelet-rich plasma, silver products, intermittent pneumatic compression therapy, electromagnetic therapy, and hyperbaric oxygen therapy. Sixteen of twenty studies compared an advanced therapy to standard therapy.

Primary Outcomes

For collagen, platelet-rich plasma, intermittent pneumatic compression therapy, and hyperbaric oxygen therapy, no eligible studies reported a significant improvement in the number of ulcers healed. Strength of evidence was low for each of those comparisons with only one trial for each advanced wound care therapy (see Executive Summary Table 2). For biological dressings, we found low strength of evidence of improved healing compared with standard care (55% versus 34% healed). The biological skin equivalent Apligraf significantly increased healed ulcers compared to compression bandaging in one trial (63% versus 49%) but the strength of evidence was low. In two trials, Dermagraft was not significantly better than compression bandaging. One trial comparing a keratinocyte product to standard care found improved healing versus standard care although a second trial found no difference. The pooled risk ratio was significant with healing in 38% versus 24% (RR=1.57, 95% CI 1.16-2.11; p=0.003). Two trials of keratinocyte therapies found no difference in ulcer healing when compared to another advanced wound care therapy. Silver creams improved healing in two studies (one comparing silver cream to standard care and one comparing silver cream to a copper-based cream) while three studies of silver dressings found mixed results (significant benefit in one study of silver dressing compared to non-silver dressing and no differences in two studies with non-silver or alternative silver dressings as the comparator). Strength of evidence was low for these outcomes. Two trials of electromagnetic therapy found mixed results; strength of evidence was low.

Few studies reported time to ulcer healing. Two studies of the biological skin equivalent Apligraf found shorter time to ulcer healing as did the study comparing a keratinocyte product to standard care. Two other keratinocyte studies reported no significant differences in time to ulcer healing as did a study comparing a silver dressing to a non-silver dressing. Strength of evidence was low for these comparisons. Two studies of silver products reported higher global assessment outcomes in the silver groups; a study of electromagnetic therapy reported no difference between groups. Only studies of electromagnetic therapy reported patient activity levels; one finding no difference between treatment groups and one noting improvements pre- to post-treatment.

Secondary Outcomes

The most commonly reported secondary outcomes were ulcers infected during treatment (8 studies), ulcer recurrence (7 studies), and pain (9 studies). The collagen treatment study reported fewer ulcers infected in the collagen group. No other study reported a difference between treatment groups. The biological dressings study reported fewer recurring ulcers in the active treatment group compared to standard care. No other differences were reported. One of the EMT studies reported a significant reduction in pain from baseline to 30 days in patients receiving EMT. Other studies reporting pain found no differences between treatment groups. No studies reported amputation, revascularization or other surgery, time to recurrence, or need for home care. Two studies reported hospitalization and one reported quality of life with no difference between treatment arms in the studies. No significant differences were observed in all-cause mortality, study withdrawals due to adverse events, or allergic reactions to treatment.

Advanced Wound Care Therapies for Non-Healing Diabetic, Venous, and Arterial Ulcers: A Systematic Review

Executive Summary Table 2. Strength of Evidence - Advanced Wound Care Therapies for Venous Ulcers

Treatment	Control(s)	Outcome	Number of Studies (n for Primary Outcome)*	Comments	Strength of Evidence
Collagen	Standard care	Percentage of ulcers healed	1 (73)	One fair quality RCT found no significant differences between treatment groups.	Low
		Mean time to ulcer healing		Outcome not reported.	Insufficient
Biological Dressings	Standard care with compression bandage	Percentage of ulcers healed	1 (120)	One fair quality study found biological dressing (OASIS) more effective at 12 weeks but not 6 months versus standard care.	Low
		Mean time to ulcer healing		Outcome not reported.	Insufficient
Biological Skin Equivalents [BSE] – Dermagraft	Standard care with compression bandage	Percentage of ulcers healed	2 (44)	Data from two small trials (fair quality) found Dermagraft was not more effective than standard care.	Low
		Mean time to ulcer healing		Outcome not reported.	Insufficient
Biological Skin Equivalents [BSE] – Apligraf	Standard care with compression bandage	Percentage of ulcers healed	1 (275)	One large fair quality trial found significant improvement with Apligraf versus standard compression therapy.	Low
		Mean time to ulcer healing		Significant improvement with Apligraf versus standard compression therapy.	Low
Keratinocyte Therapy	Standard care with compression bandage	Percentage of ulcers healed	2 (418)	Keratinocyte therapy was more effective than standard care (RR=1.57, 95% CI 1.16 to 2.11, I²=0%). The trials were rated fair quality.	Moderate
		Mean time to ulcer healing		Inconsistent results, one trial found a significant difference versus standard care and one found no difference between groups.	Low
Keratinocyte Therapy (Cryopreserved)	Advanced therapy control (Lyophilized keratinocytes)	Percentage of ulcers healed	1 (50)	One poor quality trial reported no differences between treatment groups.	Low
		Mean time to ulcer healing		No difference between groups.	Low
Keratinocyte Therapy	Advanced therapy control (Pneumatic compression)	Percentage of ulcers healed	1 (27)	One fair quality trial reported no differences between treatment groups.	Low
		Mean time to ulcer healing		Outcome not reported.	Insufficient
Platelet-Rich Plasma	Placebo	Percentage of ulcers healed	1 (86)	One fair quality trial reported no differences between treatment groups.	Low
		Mean time to ulcer healing		Outcome not reported.	Insufficient

Advanced Wound Care Therapies for Non-Healing Diabetic, Venous, and Arterial Ulcers: A Systematic Review

Treatment	Control(s)	Outcome	Number of Studies (n for Primary Outcome)*	Comments	Strength of Evidence
Silver, Dressings	Controls (non-silver dressing, ionic silver vs. lipido-colloid silver)	Percentage of ulcers healed	3 (536)	Inconsistent results from two fair quality trials, one found a significant difference versus non-silver dressing and one found no difference. One fair quality trial found no difference between two silver dressing groups.	Low
		Mean time to ulcer healing	2 (250)	Two fair quality trials; one found no significant difference between silver and non-silver dressings; one did not report significance	Low
Silver, Cream/Ointment	Controls (placebo, non-adherent dressing, standard care)	Percentage of ulcers healed	3 (199)	One fair quality trial found significant benefit compared to standard care; one fair and one good quality trail found no benefit compared to placebo or standard dressing.	Low
		Mean time to ulcer healing		Outcome not reported.	Insufficient
Silver, Cream	Placebo, tri-peptide copper cream	Percentage of ulcers healed	1 (86)	One three-armed trial of fair quality trial found silver more effective than tri-peptide copper cream but not placebo.	Low
		Mean time to ulcer healing		Outcome not reported.	Insufficient
Intermittent Pneumatic Compression (IPC)	Unna's boot dressing	Percentage of ulcers healed	1 (53)	One fair quality trial found no significant difference between groups.	Low
		Mean time to ulcer healing		Outcome not reported.	Insufficient
Electromagnetic Therapy (EMT)	Sham	Percentage of ulcers healed	2 (56)	Inconsistent results between trials. Study quality was fair.	Low
		Mean time to ulcer healing	1 (37)	Comparable between groups.	Low
Hyperbaric Oxygen Therapy (HBOT)	Sham	Percentage of ulcers healed	1 (16)	One good quality trial found no significant difference between groups.	Low
		Mean time to ulcer healing		Outcome not reported.	Insufficient

*Number of ulcers evaluated for the primary outcome.

The evidence is rated using the following grades: (1) high strength indicates further research is very unlikely to change the confidence in the estimate of effect, meaning that the evidence reflects the true effect; (2) moderate strength denotes further research may change our confidence in the estimate of effect and may change the estimate; (3) low strength indicates further research is very likely to have an important impact on the confidence in the estimate of effect and is likely to change the estimate, meaning there is low confidence that the evidence reflects the true effect; and (4) insufficient, indicating that the evidence is unavailable or does not permit a conclusion.

Key Question #3. What are the efficacy and harms of therapies for arterial ulcers? Is efficacy dependent on ancillary therapies? Does efficacy differ according to patient demographics, comorbid conditions, treatment compliance, or activity level?

We identified only one small (n=31), fair quality study of advanced wound care therapies for patients specifically identified as having arterial ulcers. This small study suggested that biological skin equivalent, may improve ulcer healing when used on ischemic foot ulcers or partial open foot amputations following revascularization surgery. At 12 weeks, healing was reported in 86% of the biological skin equivalent group and 40% of the standard care control group (p<0.01). Median time to healing was shorter in the biological skin equivalent group (7 weeks versus 15 weeks; p=0.002). Other outcomes did not differ significantly from standard care. The mean age of patients was 70 years and 75% of enrollees were men. Race/ethnicity data were not reported. Authors did not report on the effect of baseline patient characteristics, treatment compliance, or activity level on ulcer healing.

In studies of mixed ulcer types, a collagen matrix product (one fair quality study comparing collagen to standard care, n=24 randomized) improved ulcer healing (86% versus 29%, p=0.01). Improved healing was also observed in two studies of biological dressings - one fair quality study comparing biological dressing to standard care (n=50; 80% versus 65%, p<0.05), one poor quality study comparing biological dressing to another advanced wound care therapy (hyaluronic acid dressing, n=54; 81% versus 46%, p<0.001). Silver products (2 studies reporting, both fair quality and comparing a silver foam dressing to a non-silver foam dressing and a silver dressing to an advanced iodine-based dressing, n=410 randomized) and negative pressure wound therapy (1 study comparing NPWT to standard care, n=60) did not improve healing. There were mixed results for time to ulcer healing and, overall, no differences between investigational treatment and either standard care (5 studies) or another advanced care therapy (2 studies) on other outcomes. Only one study (of fair quality and comparing a silver dressing to an iodine-based advanced care dressing) looked at the effects of ulcer duration and ulcer size finding no difference in healing for ulcers of less than 12 weeks versus more than 12 weeks or ulcers of 3.6 cm^2 or less versus greater than 3.6 cm^2.

One good quality study of wounds associated with partial foot amputation (n=162) found that NPWT (compared to standard care) improved wound healing (56% versus 39%, p=0.04) and decreased mean time to healing (56 days versus 77 days, p=0.005). There were significantly more infections in the NPWT group (17% versus 6%, p=0.04), but the incidence of other adverse events did not differ between the NPWT and standard care groups. The effects of ancillary therapies, baseline characteristics, activity level and compliance were not explored.

Summary

For arterial ulcers, one small, fair quality study found that a biological skin equivalent, may improve the incidence and rate of complete ulcer healing when used on ischemic foot ulcers following revascularization surgery. Other outcomes did not differ significantly from standard care. The effects of ancillary therapies or baseline patient characteristics were not explored in the study. We found no RCTs that included any of the other therapies of interest exclusively in patients with arterial lower extremity ulcers.

In seven studies of mixed ulcer types, collagen and biological dressings were found to improve ulcer healing; silver products and negative pressure wound therapy did not. There were mixed results for time to ulcer healing and, overall, no differences between investigational treatment and control on other outcomes. The studies were of poor to fair quality.

One good quality study of ulcers associated with partial foot amputation showed a benefit of NPWT with respect to healed ulcers and mean time to healing. There were significantly more infections in the NPWT group but the incidence of other adverse events did not differ between the NPWT and standard care groups.

DISCUSSION

Chronic lower extremity ulcers are a common and serious health problem. A wide range of standard treatment approaches to achieve ulcer healing are used (e.g., off-loading, compression, leg elevation, etc.) based on patient and ulcer factors and provider preferences. While many ulcers heal completely within several weeks, a significant portion either do not heal or increase in size, depth, and severity. These chronic ulcers can result in considerable clinical morbidity and health care costs.

Many types of advanced wound care therapies exist but all represent considerably greater product costs compared to standard therapy. These costs may be justified if they result in improved ulcer healing, reduced morbidity, fewer lower extremity amputations, and improved patient functional status. In addition to the treatment selected, many potential factors contribute to the success or failure of the ulcer healing process including ulcer etiology; ulcer area, depth, duration, and location; patient comorbid conditions; and patient compliance with the treatment protocol. Much of the existing research on advanced wound care therapies has attempted to minimize the influence of many of these factors by limiting enrollment to patients with ulcers of a particular size, including only patients with adequate circulation, and excluding patients taking certain classes of medications. Furthermore, many of the trials are industry sponsored (55% of the studies included in our review) and the role of the sponsor is typically not stated, definitions of "chronic" ulcers vary widely, and few studies are of sufficient duration to assess whether healing is maintained.

Our systematic review of randomized controlled trials found discouragingly low strength evidence regarding the effectiveness and comparative effectiveness of advanced wound care therapies for treatment of lower extremity ulcers. This was primarily due to the fact that for each ulcer type (diabetic, venous, or arterial) individual categories of advanced wound care therapies were only evaluated in a few studies, often in highly selected populations, and frequently had conflicting findings. Furthermore, within each category of wound care therapies several different types of interventions were used making it difficult to determine if results were replicable in other studies or generalizable to broader clinical settings. Additionally, most studies compared advanced wound care therapies to standard care or placebo. Therefore there is little comparative effectiveness research evaluating one advanced wound care therapy to another. It has been noted that standard care is an inappropriate comparator for studies of advanced therapy since patients have likely already failed standard care. For arterial ulcers we identified only a single study of any advanced wound care therapy (and this was compared to standard care) despite the clinical importance of arterial ulcers.

However, based on the available findings we conclude that for patients with diabetic chronic ulcers, there is moderate strength of evidence that the biological skin equivalent Apligraf and negative pressure wound therapy improve healing compared to standard care. There is low strength evidence that advanced wound care therapies improved the percentage of ulcers healed compared to standard care for the following therapies: collagen (notably Graftjacket), the biological skin equivalent Dermagraft, platelet-derived growth factors, silver cream, and hyperbaric oxygen therapy but results were not uniform for any treatment group. Most beneficial effects were derived from single or few studies so we recommend caution regarding translating these findings of effectiveness into broader clinical application. Pooled analyses were possible for several therapies and demonstrated a significant improvement in ulcer healing compared to standard care for Apligraf (a biological skin equivalent), platelet-derived growth factors, and negative pressure wound therapy; no improvement was observed for Dermagraft (a biological skin equivalent). Few studies compared one advanced treatment to another but in those studies, no differences in percentage of ulcers healed were found between the two treatment arms. For time to ulcer healing, the pattern of findings was similar and strength of evidence was low for all treatment comparisons reporting that outcome. No studies reported a significant difference in adverse events for any treatment comparison.

Findings for venous ulcers were similar. Although some individual trials of biological dressings (notably OASIS), biological skin equivalents (Apligraf), keratinocytes, silver cream and dressing, and electromagnetic therapy noted significant benefit of the therapy in percentage of ulcers healed compared to standard care, overall the results for each therapy were mixed. In pooled analyses only keratinocytes resulted in significantly better healing compared to standard care. Strength of evidence was moderate for the benefit of keratinocyte therapy and low for the other therapies. Few studies of venous ulcers compared two advanced therapies and, where reported, typically found no differences. Time to ulcer healing was reported infrequently. No advanced wound care therapy was observed to result in an increase in adverse events.

We identified only one study of patients with arterial ulcers despite the clinical importance of this population. It is possible that patients with arterial disease were included in the studies of diabetic ulcers or venous ulcers (i.e., mixed etiology). In one study of patients with non-healing lower extremity ulcers or amputation wounds following a revascularization procedure, Apligraf increased ulcer healing and decreased time to healing compared to standard care with no difference in adverse events.

For amputation wounds, one study of negative pressure wound therapy versus standard care found significantly better healing with no difference in adverse events.

Despite finding benefits of some therapies compared to standard care, the methodological quality of individual studies reviewed was predominantly fair or poor. Common factors limiting the quality were inadequate allocation concealment, no blinding (including no blinding of outcome assessment), failure to use intention-to-treat analysis methods, and failure to adequately describe study dropouts and withdrawals. With methodological flaws, few trials reporting, and heterogeneity in the comparators, study duration, and how outcomes were assessed, the overall strength of evidence was low. While a wide range of patients were enrolled in studies most were older than age 60 years, male, of white race, likely compliant with treatment protocols, and possessed ulcers that were relatively small as measured by surface area. However, authors rarely reported outcomes by patient demographic, comorbidity or ulcer characteristics. Therefore, we found insufficient evidence to guide clinicians and policy makers regarding whether efficacy differs according to patient demographics, comorbid conditions, treatment compliance, or activity level.

APPLICABILITY AND COST EFFECTIVENESS

It is not well known how outcomes reported in studies of selected populations will translate to daily practice settings including in Veterans Health Administration facilities. There is evidence of good success in ulcer healing with strict adherence to off-loading for diabetic ulcers and compression therapy for venous ulcers. The patients enrolled in trials were likely more compliant than typical patients and received very close monitoring. Therefore, results from these studies may overestimate benefits and underestimate harms in non-study populations.

Our review was limited to studies of FDA approved products. We excluded studies with wounds of multiple etiologies (e.g., vascular, pressure, trauma, surgery) if they did not report results by etiology. We also excluded studies if they did not report our primary outcomes of healed wounds or time to complete healing. Many studies report change in ulcer size but the clinical benefit of change in ulcer size has not been established.

Furthermore, we did not conduct cost effectiveness analyses or assess additional costs of care associated with chronic ulcers. Despite the high costs of advanced wound care therapies it is possible that they may be cost effective or even cost saving if found to improve ulcer healing; reduce ulcer associated morbidity, hospitalizations, medical care and amputations; and improve functional status and quality of life. Based on our findings from randomized controlled trials the decision of if, when, and in whom to use advanced wound care therapies as well as the type of advanced wound care therapy selected is difficult. Additionally, because little comparative effectiveness research exists to guide choices, decisions may be based on other factors including wound care product cost, ease of use, and patient and provider preferences (the latter also influenced by personal experience with ulcer and patient characteristics).

FUTURE RESEARCH

Our review highlights several much needed areas for future research. Most studies compared an advanced therapy to either standard ulcer care or placebo treatment. Few studies (10 of the 35 eligible studies of diabetic ulcers, 4 of the 20 eligible studies of venous ulcers, and none for arterial or mixed ulcers) directly compared two advanced therapies. Furthermore, few studies provided a run-in period with carefully monitored standard care to exclude patients for whom carefully monitored standard care would obviate the need for advanced therapy. Therefore, additional randomized trials of advanced wound care therapies versus standard care are needed to replicate or refute current findings. Comparative effectiveness research is also needed to evaluate the relative benefits and harms of different advanced wound care therapies. In both effectiveness and comparative effectiveness research, the sample sizes should be adequate to report specific outcome reporting according to key patient and ulcer characteristics including age, race, gender, and ulcer size, location, and depth. We note below the limitations of the existing research by type of ulcer and therapy assessed.

Of the studies of diabetic ulcers included in this review, only two focused on biological dressings (using different products) and two on platelet-rich plasma. We identified no studies of topical oxygen or electromagnetic therapy. No studies reported on return to daily activities or the need for home care related to ulcer treatment and only one study reported quality of life or hospitalization. The need for amputation or revascularization and the incidence of and time to ulcer recurrence require further investigation. The majority of studies described the ulcers as diabetic foot ulcers with only six providing greater detail about ulcer location. Future research should report healing by ulcer location. Future research should also examine microvascular disease to more clearly distinguish diabetic ulcers from arterial ulcers.

For venous ulcers, we identified only one study of the following advanced wound care therapies: collagen, biological dressings, platelet rich plasma, intermittent pneumatic compression, and hyperbaric oxygen therapy. There were no studies of platelet-derived growth factors or typical oxygen. We found no studies that reported on amputations, time to ulcer recurrence, or need for home health care related to the ulcer. One study reported hospitalization, one study reported quality of life, and two studies reported return to work or daily activities.

We identified only one study of patients with arterial disease requiring advanced wound care following revascularization. Only this study and one other included patients with partial foot amputations with delayed healing. Neither of these studies reported on return to daily activities, pain, quality of life, or need for home health assistance related to the wound. There is a paucity of research on advanced wound care therapies in patients with strictly arterial disease.

In addition to specific topics needing further research, several organizations have outlined overall methodological standards for future research of wound healing therapies. The standards focus on study design, patient population, comparators, outcomes and outcome assessment, and potential sources of bias. Randomized trials, with allocation concealment and, at a minimum, blinding of third-party outcomes assessors, are recommended. The patient population should be appropriate for the treatment being studied and exclusion criteria should be minimal to enhance generalizability. Endpoints should be selected based on the purpose of the intervention (i.e., closure versus preparation for surgery) and adequate follow-up should be included to confirm healing. Dropouts and study withdrawals should be documented, including withdrawals due to ulcer deterioration. Additional research, conducted in accordance with the standards, is needed to establish the safety and efficacy of advanced wound care therapies. Finally, future research is needed to determine the effectiveness, comparative effectiveness and harms of advanced wound care therapies as used in general clinical practice settings (e.g., vascular and dermatology clinics) where patients may have more severe and larger ulcers, greater comorbidities, or increased difficulty with treatment compliance.

ABBREVIATIONS TABLE

ABI	Ankle-Brachial Index
ARD	Absolute Risk difference
BD	Biological Dressing
BMI	Body Mass Index
BSE	Biological Skin Equivalent
CI	Confidence Interval
CMS	Centers for Medicare and Medicaid Services
Col	Collagen
EMT	Electromagnetic Therapy
EST	Extracorporeal Shock Wave Therapy
FDA	Food and Drug Administration
HbA_1c	Hemoglobin A_1c
HBOT	Hyperbaric Oxygen Therapy
IPC	Intermittent Pneumatic Compression
NPWT	Negative Pressure Wound Therapy
PAD/PVD	Peripheral Artery Disease or Peripheral Vascular Disease
PDGF	Platelet-derived Growth Factor
PPP	Platelet-Poor Plasma
PRP	Platelet Rich Plasma
RCT	Randomized Controlled Trial
RR	Risk Ratio
VA	Veterans Affairs
VAMC	VA Medical Center

EVIDENCE REPORT

INTRODUCTION

Chronic ulcers (i.e., ulcers that are unresponsive to initial therapy or that persist despite appropriate care) are estimated to affect over 6 million people in the United States.[1] The incidence is expected to increase as the population ages and as the number of individuals with diabetes increases.[1] Chronic ulcers negatively affect the quality of life and productivity of the patient and represent a financial burden to the health care system.[1,2,3] Within the Veterans Health Administration, during fiscal year 2011, there were over 227,000 ulcer encounters (inpatient and outpatient) involving over 54,000 patients and nearly 77,000 new ulcers.(Source: PAVE ProClarity Cubes (Prevention of Amputations in Veterans Every ProClarity Cubes)).

We focus on chronic ulcers of the lower extremity, in particular, ulcers attributed to either diabetes, venous disease, or arterial disease. Because advanced wound care therapies are typically used for ulcer healing following amputation, we also included post-amputation wounds. Identifying the ulcer etiology is important because the correct diagnosis is one factor in determining appropriate wound care interventions.[4] Treatment modalities and wound care therapies are also selected based on patient factors, past treatment, and provider choice. A brief description of each ulcer type is provided below. We recognize that a non-healing ulcer is likely a result of multiple factors and comorbid conditions. We categorize included studies as diabetic, venous, or arterial according to the study author's description of the ulcer type.

ULCER TYPES

Diabetic Ulcers

Approximately 15% to 25% of individuals with diabetes develop a foot ulcer at some point in their lifetime and an estimated 12% of those patients require lower extremity amputation.[1] Diabetic foot ulcers account for nearly 2/3 of all nontraumatic amputations.[4] Ulcer healing is complicated by diabetic neuropathy, decreased cellular synthesis, and susceptability to infection.[5] Neuropathy can be categorized as sensory (loss of protective sensation), motor (the anatomic structure of foot is deformed creating areas where pressure from an ill-fitting shoe can create ulcers), or autonomic (resulting in denervation of sweat glands so the skin becomes dry and cracked predisposing the foot to infection, calluses etc.).[3,4] Diabetic ulcers are typically located on the plantar aspect of the foot, over the metatarsal heads, or under the heel.[6] The ulcers are characterized by even wound margins, a deep wound bed, cellulitis or underlying osteomyelitis, granular tissue (unless peripheral vascular disease is also present), and low to moderate drainage.[6] Patients should be assessed for adequacy of circulation (claudication or extremity pain at rest, diminished or absent pulses, cool temperature, pallor on elevation, ABI), although due to issues with non-compressible vessels, toe pressures, ultrasonography, or other noninvasive vascular studies may be needed.[7] Diabetic ulcers are typically graded using the Wagner[8] classification:

> Grade 0 – no open lesions in a high-risk foot
> Grade 1 – superficial ulcer involving full skin thickness but not underlying tissue

Grade 2 – deeper ulcer; penetrating to tendon, bone, or joint capsule

Grade 3 – deeper ulcer with cellulitis or abscess formation, often with osteomyelitis or tendinitis

Grade 4 – localized gangrene

Grade 5 – extensive gangrene involving the whole foot

The University of Texas Diabetic Wound Classification System is also used.[9] This system incorporates ischemia and infection in ulcer assessment. Standard treatment for Grade 1 and 2 diabetic ulcers includes debridement of necrotic tissue, infection control, local ulcer care (keeping the ulcer clean and moist but free of excess fluids), mechanical off-loading, management of blood glucose levels, and education on foot care.[4,7] Osteomyelitis is a serious complication and a delay in diagnosis is associated with significant morbidity (e.g., non-healing, ulcer sepsis, limb loss).[5]

Venous Leg Ulcers

The most common cause of lower extremity ulcers is venous insufficiency. This accounts for 70-90% of leg ulcers.[1,5] The ulcers develop within the setting of venous hypertension; elevated pressures are most commonly caused by valvular incompetence and result in an inefficient return of venous blood upon muscle contraction. Although a number of initiating factors may lead to the valvular incompetence of deep or perforating veins (e.g., deep vein thrombosis, phlebitis, trauma, surgery, or obesity), the resulting clinical picture of chronic venous insufficiency is the same. The congested vessels and pooling of blood result in increased vascular permeability. Water, proteins, and red blood cells leak out into the interstitial space, and pericapillary fibrin deposition occurs. This results in the symptoms of leg edema, hyperpigmentation (from extravasation of red blood cells and hemosiderin buildup), and lipodermosclerosis. Ulcers are thought to develop in this setting of venous stasis for a number of reasons: pericapillary fibrin deposits limit diffusion of oxygen and nutrients to skin tissue; leaked extravascular proteins may trap growth factors and matrix materials necessary for preventing and repairing the breakdown of tissue; and the accumulation or "trapping" of white blood cells may cause the release of proteolytic enzymes and inflammatory mediators.[10] Venous ulcers occur most commonly in the leg (compared with the foot predominance of arterial and diabetic ulcers) and are characteristically found over the medial malleolus. These ulcers are often shallow and can be very large relative to other types of ulcers.[11] Standard treatment is centered on the use of mechanical compression and limb elevation to reverse tissue edema and improve venous blood flow by increasing the hydrostatic pressure.[12]

Arterial Leg Ulcers

Ulcers associated with peripheral artery disease, also commonly known as ischemic ulcers, account for approximately 10% of lower extremity ulcers.[3] This ulcer type develops due to arterial occlusion, which limits the blood supply and results in ischemia and necrosis of tissue in the supplied area. This occlusion is most commonly from atherosclerotic disease, so major risk factors for ischemic ulcers are the same as those in peripheral arterial disease (PAD); cigarette smoking, diabetes, hyperlipidemia, and hypertension.[3] Similarly, patients with ischemic ulcers will complain of PAD-related symptoms such as intermittent claudication or pain that continues despite leg elevation. Other signs of decreased limb perfusion may also be present, such as a shiny, atrophic appearance of the skin, diminished leg hair, cold feet, and dystrophic nails.[4,6]

Evidence of diminished arterial blood flow may be established by finding diminished or absent pedal pulses or, most importantly, by measuring an ankle-brachial index (ABI).[4,5] Because ischemic ulcers are related to poor perfusion, they typically occur at the most distal sites (e.g., the tips of toes) or in areas of increased pressure (e.g., over bony prominences). These painful ulcers often present as well-demarcated, deep lesions, giving the lesions a classically described "punched-out" appearance.[5] Care for ischemic ulcers is centered on reestablishing blood flow and minimizing further losses of perfusion. With severe ischemia, the primary methods for achieving this are vascular surgery and lifestyle modifications. It is important to avoid treatment with mechanical compression if arterial occlusion is a contributing source for the development of an ulcer, as this leads to a worsening of tissue ischemia and necrosis.[4]

ADVANCED WOUND CARE THERAPIES

If ulcers do not adequately heal with standard treatment, additional modalities may be required. We define advanced wound care therapies as interventions used when standard wound care has failed. A large and growing array of advanced wound care therapies of different composition and indications have been developed though their efficacy, comparative effectiveness and harm is not well established. Therapies included in this review are: collagen products (COL), biological dressings (BD), biological skin equivalents (BSE), keratinocytes, platelet-derived growth factor (PDGF), platelet-rich plasma (PRP), silver products, intermittent pneumatic compression therapy (IPC), negative pressure wound therapy (NPWT), electromagnetic therapy (EMT), hyperbaric oxygen (HBOT), topical oxygen, and ozone oxygen. Because collagen may be a vehicle to deliver other bioactive ingredients, we have included in the collagen section only studies of collagen as a matrix material.

A complete description of these therapies, including reference citations, is presented in Appendix A; a brief description follows.

Collagen: Naturally occurring proteins known as collagens have diverse roles in ulcer healing including 1) acting as a substrate for hemostasis, 2) chemotactic properties that attract granulocytes, macrophages, and fibroblasts to aid healing, 3) providing a scaffold for more rapid transition to mature collagen production and alignment, or 4) providing a template for cellular attachment, migration, and proliferation.

Biological Dressings: These dressings consist of biomaterials made from various components of the extracellular matrix and are theorized to stimulate ulcer healing by providing a structural scaffold and the growth signals important to complex cellular interactions within ulcers, both of which are dysfunctional and contribute to the persistence of chronic ulcers.

Biological Skin Equivalents: These products are laboratory-derived tissue constructs, designed to resemble various layers of real human skin. They are thought to increase healing by stimulating fibrovascular ingrowth and epithelialization of host tissues.

Keratinocytes: Keratinocyte-based therapies for wound healing exist in a variety of forms and are proposed to work by stimulating proliferation and migration of host epithelium from wound edges through the production of growth factors and other cytokines.

<u>Platelet-Derived Growth Factors</u>: These products are designed to help repair and replace dead skin and other tissues by attracting cells that repair wounds and helping to close and heal the ulcers.

<u>Platelet-Rich Plasma</u>: Plasma with a high platelet concentration aids wound healing by attracting undifferentiated cells and activating cell division.

<u>Silver Products</u>: Multiple silver-based products have been developed to aid wound healing due to their broad bactericidal action. Cytotoxicity to host cells, including keratinocytes and fibroblasts, may delay wound closure.

<u>Intermittent Pneumatic Compression</u>: Delivered through inflatable garments containing one or more air chambers, compression propels deep venous blood towards the heart. This treatment benefits the non-ambulatory patient by increasing blood flow velocity in the deep veins and reducing stasis, decreasing venous hypertension, flushing valve pockets, and decreasing interstitial edema.

<u>Negative Pressure Wound Therapy</u>: This therapy involves creating a tightly sealed dressing around a wound and using a suction pump to apply negative pressure evenly across the surface in a continuous or intermittent manner. This process is proposed to enhance wound healing by increasing granulation tissue and local perfusion, reducing tissue edema, decreasing bacterial load, and stimulating cellular proliferation via induction of mechanical stress.

<u>Electromagnetic Therapy</u>: This process uses the electrical field that develops from exposure to an oscillating magnetic field. The treatment is thought to work by mimicking or enhancing natural wound-induced electrical fields produced in normal human skin.

<u>Hyperbaric Oxygen Therapy</u>: This therapy requires specialized compression chambers capable of delivering increased concentrations of oxygen (usually 100% oxygen) under elevated atmospheric pressures. Many key aspects of ulcer healing are oxygen dependent and raising arterial oxygen tension and the blood-oxygen level delivered to a chronic ulcer is thought to supply a missing nutrient, promote the oxygen dependent steps in ulcer healing, up regulate local growth factors, and down regulate inhibitory cytokines.

<u>Topical Oxygen Therapy</u>: These products aim to promote ulcer healing by correcting the low oxygen levels found within chronic ulcer.

<u>Ozone Oxygen Therapy</u>: Ozone is an oxidizing agent theorized to promote tissue healing by assisting in the destruction of defective cells, bacteria, and viruses.

PURPOSE AND SCOPE OF REVIEW

A large and growing array of advanced wound care therapies of different composition and for different indications has been developed though the effectiveness, comparative effectiveness, and potential harm is not well established. The purpose of this review is to synthesize the evidence on advanced wound care therapies for treatment of non-healing diabetic, venous, and arterial lower extremity ulcers. We focus on FDA-approved therapies used in adult patients. Our outcomes of interest are complete healing and time to complete healing. Secondary outcomes and adverse events are also reported.

METHODS

TOPIC DEVELOPMENT

This project was nominated by Rajiv Jain, MD (Chief Consultant, Office of Patient Care Services) and Jeffrey Robbins, DPM (Director, Podiatry Service). Our key questions were developed with input from a technical expert panel. We also received guidance from Carolyn Robinson, NP, MSN, and Eric Affeldt, DPM, both from the Minneapolis VA Health Care System.

We address the following key questions:

1. What are the efficacy and harms of therapies for diabetic ulcers? Is efficacy dependent on ancillary therapies? Does efficacy differ according to patient demographics, comorbid conditions, treatment compliance, or activity level?

2. What are the efficacy and harms of therapies for venous ulcers? Is efficacy dependent on ancillary therapies? Does efficacy differ according to patient demographics, comorbid conditions, treatment compliance, or activity level?

3. What are the efficacy and harms of therapies for arterial ulcers? Is efficacy dependent on ancillary therapies? Does efficacy differ according to patient demographics, comorbid conditions, treatment compliance, or activity level?

SEARCH STRATEGY

We searched MEDLINE (Ovid) for randomized controlled trials (RCTs) published from 1995 to August 2012 using standard search terms. We limited the search to articles with adults and published in the English language. Search terms included: skin ulcer, foot ulcer, leg ulcer, varicose ulcer, diabetic ulcer, diabetic foot, wound healing, venous insufficiency, artificial skin, biological dressings, negative-pressure wound therapy, collagen, silver, topical oxygen, hyperbaric oxygen, electromagnetic, platelet-derived growth factor, platelet-rich plasma, and intermittent pneumatic compression devices. The search strategy is presented in Appendix B.

We did a similar search of the Cochrane Library, and obtained additional articles by a hand-search of reference lists of pertinent studies and systematic reviews and suggestions from members of our technical expert panel.

STUDY SELECTION

Titles and abstracts were reviewed by researchers trained in the critical analysis of literature. Full text versions of potentially eligible articles were retrieved for review. Our inclusion criteria were as follows:

- Randomized controlled trials
- Studies reported in the English language
- Studies involving adults (18 years and older)

- Intervention must involve collagen-based products, biologic dressings, biologic skin equivalents, keratinocytes, platelet-derived growth factors, platelet-rich plasma, silver products, intermittent pneumatic compression therapy, negative pressure wound therapy, electromagnetic therapy, or hyperbaric or topical oxygen
- Study reports patient outcomes of interest (healed ulcers or time to healing)
- Study published in a peer-reviewed publication after 1995

DATA ABSTRACTION

We abstracted the following data for each included study: author, date of publication, country where study was conducted, funding source, Therapy type, sample characteristics (gender, age, race/ethnicity, body mass index [BMI], hemoglobin A_1c [HbA_1c], smoking status, work days missed, ankle-brachial index [ABI]), ulcer characteristics (type, size, location, grade, duration, infection status), comorbid conditions (hypertension, peripheral vascular disease [PVD], cardiovascular disease, diabetes, or amputation), study inclusion and exclusion criteria, treatment groups, intervention characteristics (product descriptions and application frequency/ duration), treatment duration, follow-up duration, study withdrawals, treatment compliance and study quality (allocation concealment, blinding, analysis approach, description of withdrawals). We abstracted primary outcomes (ulcers healed, time to complete ulcer closure, patient global assessment, and return to daily activities) and secondary outcomes (ulcer infection, amputation, revascularization surgery, ulcer recurrence, time to ulcer recurrence, pain or discomfort, hospitalizations, need for home care, quality of life, all-cause mortality, study withdrawals due to adverse events, and allergic reactions to treatment), by ulcer type, for each treatment. We assessed outcomes following treatment and at follow-up, or as reported. All abstraction was done by trained research personnel and verified by a second research associate under the supervision of a Principal Investigator.

QUALITY ASSESSMENT

We assessed the quality of studies pertaining to the key questions. Individual randomized studies were rated as good, fair, or poor quality based the following criteria: allocation concealment, blinding, analysis approach, and description of withdrawals – a modification of the Cochrane approach to determining risk of bias.[13] We assessed studies for applicability to U.S. Veterans.

DATA SYNTHESIS

We constructed evidence tables showing the study characteristics and results for all included studies, organized by key question and intervention. We critically analyzed studies to compare their characteristics, methods, and findings. We compiled a summary of findings for each key question or clinical topic, and drew conclusions based on qualitative synthesis of the findings. Where feasible, results were pooled.

RATING THE BODY OF EVIDENCE

We assessed the overall strength of evidence using the method reported by Owens et al.[14] The overall evidence was rated as: (1) high, meaning high confidence that the evidence reflects the true effect; (2) moderate, indicating moderate confidence that further research may change our confidence in the estimate of effect and may change the estimate; (3) low, meaning there is low confidence that the evidence reflects the true effect; or (4) insufficient, indicating that evidence either is unavailable or does not permit a conclusion.

PEER REVIEW

A draft version of this report was reviewed by clinical content experts as well as clinical leadership. Their comments and our responses are presented in Appendix C.

RESULTS

LITERATURE FLOW

We reviewed 1,230 titles and abstracts from the electronic searches. After applying inclusion/
exclusion criteria at the abstract level 1,053 references were excluded. We retrieved 177 full-
text articles for further review and another 130 references were excluded leaving 47 included
references. We added 21 articles from reviewing reference lists of relevant articles and
systematic reviews for a total of 68 articles on 64 trials. We grouped the studies by ulcer etiology
to address our key questions (see Figure 1).

Figure 1. Literature Flow Diagram

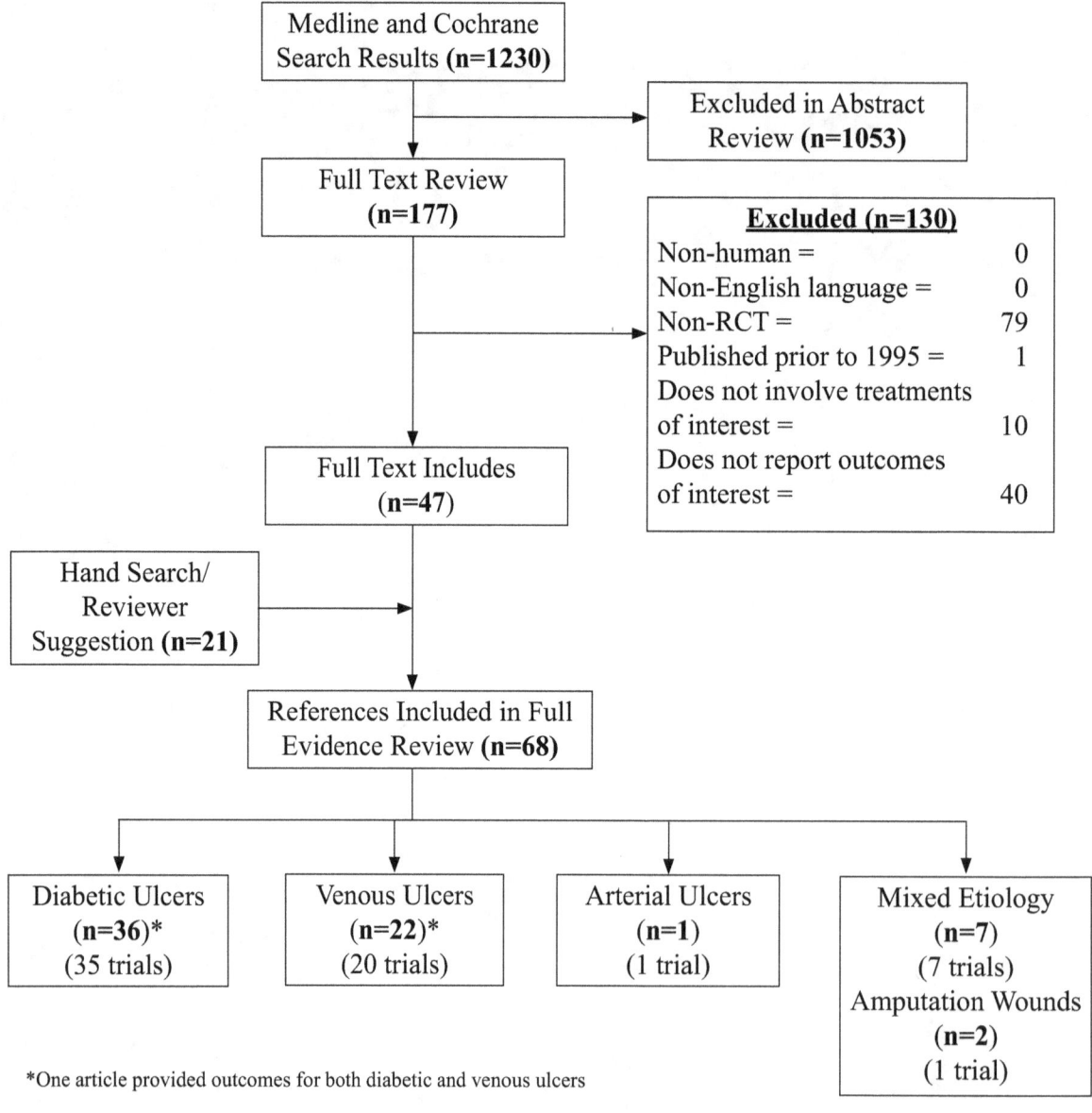

*One article provided outcomes for both diabetic and venous ulcers

KEY QUESTION #1. What are the efficacy and harms of therapies for diabetic ulcers? Is efficacy dependent on ancillary therapies? Does efficacy differ according to patient demographics, comorbid conditions, treatment compliance, or activity level?

Overview of Studies

Table 1 contains an overview of studies of treatments for diabetic ulcers.[15-50] Thirty-six articles (35 trials) met eligibility criteria including 4 trials of collagen (n=489 randomized), 2 trials of biological dressings (n=124), 7 trials of biological skin equivalents (one trial included a biological dressing arm) (n=989), 9 trials (in 10 articles) of platelet-derived growth factors (one trial included a biological dressing arm) (n=990), 2 trials of platelet-rich plasma (n=96), 4 trials of silver products (n=280), 3 trials of negative pressure wound therapy (n=418), 5 trials of hyperbaric oxygen therapy (n=326), and 1 trial of ozone-oxygen therapy (n=61). Twenty-five trials compared an advanced wound care therapy to standard care or placebo. In nine trials, the comparator was a different advanced therapy. One trial included both comparators.

Overall, the mean age of study participants ranged from 51 to 71 years; in the majority of studies the mean age was between 55 and 65 years. Between 28% and 100% were male although in all but 3 studies, 60% or more were male. Few studies reported race. In those reporting, 58% to 86% were white, 8% to 16% were black, 6% to 30% were Hispanic, and 2% to 12% were Native American. Mean ulcer sizes ranged from 1.9 to 41.5 cm², however, the mean ulcer size was greater than 10 cm² in only 6 of 29 studies reporting. Mean ulcer durations ranged from 14.5 days to 21.6 months with durations of greater than 1 year in 6 of 21 studies reporting.

In 26 trials the ulcer was described as a "foot" ulcer, in 7 trials the ulcer was described as a "lower extremity" ulcer, and in 2 trials ulcer was described only as a "diabetic ulcer." Of the "foot" ulcer trials, 7 provided more detail. Three trials included only plantar ulcers and 1 included only calcaneal, dorsal, and plantar ulcers. In 1 trial, 38% of ulcers were located on the toes and 39% on the heel, in a second trial, 68% were plantar and 32% were non-plantar, and in third trial 61% were on the heel and sole and 39% were on the toes. The ulcer type was further described as neuropathic in 11 trials, ischemic in 1 trial, neuroischemic in 1 trial, and mixed in 3 trials. Of the remaining trials, 16 had inclusion criteria related to adequate circulation or exclusion criteria related to severe arterial disease and 3 did not specify criteria related to circulation.

Collagen

Four randomized controlled trials with a total enrollment of 489 patients compared the efficacy of collagen to standard care for the treatment of diabetic ulcers.[15-18] Three of the trials described the ulcers as "foot" ulcers; one included lower extremity and foot ulcers.[15] A fifth trial of 19 patients with type 2 diabetes and chronic diabetic foot lesions randomized participants to collagen or to standard care.[51] The focus of this trial was on changes to biomarkers over 5 days of treatment. The authors did report that, at a mean treatment duration of 26 days, 8 of 13 patients treated with collagen (62%) achieved wound closure. In the standard care group, no wound closure was observed and after a mean of 19 days, patients received a different treatment (not specified). Due to the incomplete reporting, we have not included this study in the summary of collagen trials (below).

The four included studies were conducted in the United States and industry funded. Study quality was rated fair for all trials. Participants had mean age of 57 years; 74 percent were male (Table 2). Collagen trial durations were eight[17] and twelve weeks.[15,16,18] The studies included non-healing diabetic ulcers of at least four weeks in duration. One study included a 2 week run-in with standard care (debridement, moist dressings, and off-loading) and excluded individuals with a greater than 30% decrease in ulcer size during the run-in period.[15] Inclusion criteria allowed for all ulcers greater than 1.0 cm^2, and the average enrolled ulcer size was 3.1 cm^2. None of the trials reported a difference between treatment arms in ulcer size or ulcer duration. Infected ulcers were excluded from all studies and use of antibiotics during the trial was not reported to be on an "as needed" basis in one trial. In all trials, adequate circulation was required for inclusion. Standard care included off-loading in all trials with one study reporting asking about compliance with off-loading at each visit. Compliance with therapy was reported to be greater than 90% in one study (patients kept a diary of dressing changes).[16] Two studies excluded patients for non-compliance but did not report how that was determined.[15,18] The fourth study did not report compliance.[17] One of the trials included a second intervention arm with a non-FDA approved product.[15] Results from that treatment arm are not reported. A complete summary of patient demographics and ulcer characteristics is presented in Appendix D, Table 1.

Primary Outcomes (Appendix D, Table 2)

All studies reported the percentage of ulcers healed by study completion. One study (n=86) found collagen (Graftjacket) to significantly improve ulcer healing compared to standard care (70% versus 46%; ARD=23%, 95% CI 3% to 44%).[18] The difference was maintained after adjusting for baseline ulcer size. There was no significant difference in the percentage of healed ulcers with Promogran (37% versus 28%),[16] Fibracol (48% versus 36%),[17] or formulated collagen gel (45% versus 31%)[15] compared to standard care. One study reported a trend toward a higher percentages of ulcers healed in ulcers of less than 6 months duration (45% versus 33%, p=0.06); ulcer size (<10 cm^2 versus ≥10 cm^2) was not a factor.[16] Two studies found no difference between collagen and standard care in time to complete healing[17,18] while in a third study, time to healing was significantly shorter in patients receiving standard care (7.0 weeks versus 5.8 weeks, p<0.0001).[16]

Advanced Wound Care Therapies for Non-Healing Diabetic, Venous, and Arterial Ulcers: A Systematic Review

Table 1. Overview of Therapies for Diabetic Ulcers

Study, year	N Randomized	Treatment	Product	Comparator	Healed ulcers	Mean time to ulcer healing	Global assessment	Return to daily activities	Ulcers infected during treatment	Amputation	Revascularization/surgery	Recurrence	Time to recurrence	Pain/discomfort	Hospitalization	Required home care	Quality of life	Withdrawals due to adverse events	Patients with ≥ 1 adverse event	All-cause mortality	Allergic reactions to treatment
Blume 2011[15]	52	Col	Formulated Collagen Gel	Standard	·				·									·			
Veves 2002[16]	276	Col	Promogran	Standard	·	→			·										·	·	
Donaghue 1998[17]	75	Col	Fibracol	Standard	·	·			·									·			
Reyzelman 2009[18]	86	Col	Graftjacket	Standard	+	·			·	·	·							·	·	·	
Niezgoda 2005[19]	98	BD, PDGF	OASIS	PDGF (becaplermin)	·	·						·		±					·		
Landsman 2008[20]	26	BD, BSE	OASIS	Dermagraft	·	·															
Gentzkow 1996[21]	50	BSE	Dermagraft	Standard	+	·			·			·							·		·
Naughton 1997[22]	281	BSE	Dermagraft	Standard	·	±			·			·	±						·		
Marston 2003[23]	245	BSE	Dermagraft	Standard	+	+			·	+	·										
Veves 2001[24]	277	BSE	Apligraf (Graftskin)	Standard	+	+			·										·		
Edmonds 2009[25]	82	BSE	Apligraf	Standard	+	+			·	·		·						·	·		·
DiDomenico 2011[26]	28	BSE	Apligraf	Theraskin	·	·			·	+											
Aminian 2000[27]	9	PDGF	Autologous platelet extract	Silver sulfadiazine	·	±				·											
Agrawal 2009[28]	28	PDGF	rhPDGF	Placebo gel	+	+														·	
Hardikar 2005[29]	113	PDGF	rhPDGF	Placebo gel	+	+													·		
Bhansali 2009[30]	20	PDGF	rhPDGF	Standard	·																
Wieman 1998[31]	382	PDGF	Regranex (2 doses)	Placebo gel	+	+			·			·		·				·	·		
Niezgoda 2005 See BD studies above[19]	98	PDGF	Becaplermin	Biologic dressing (OASIS)	·	·			·			·		±				·	·		
Jaiswal 2010[32]	50	PDGF	rhPDGF	Inactive gel	·																·
Steed 1995, 2006[33,34]	118	PDGF	rhPDGF	Placebo gel	+	+						·	±	·					·	·	
d'Hemecourt 1998[35]	172	PDGF	Becaplermin gel	NaCMC gel or standard care	+ vs std*	·			·					·				·	·	·	

33

Advanced Wound Care Therapies for Non-Healing Diabetic, Venous, and Arterial Ulcers: A Systematic Review

Study, year	N Randomized	Treatment	Product	Comparator	Healed ulcers	Mean time to ulcer healing	Global assessment	Return to daily activities	Ulcers infected during treatment	Amputation	Revascularization/ surgery	Recurrence	Time to recurrence	Pain/discomfort	Hospitalization	Required home care	Quality of life	Withdrawals due to adverse events	Patients with ≥ 1 adverse event	All-cause mortality	Allergic reactions to treatment
Saad Setta 2011[36]	24	PRP	PRP	Platelet poor plasma	-	+															
Driver 2006[37]	72	PRP	AutoloGel	Placebo gel	-	-						-							-	-	
Belcaro 2010[38]	66	Silver Ointment	Aidance	Standard	+																
Jacobs 2008[39]	40	Oak Bark Extract	Bensal HP	Silver cream	-														-		-
Jude 2007[40]	134	Silver Dressing	AQUA-CEL	Calcium dressing	-	-	-		-			-						-	-	-	
Viswanathan 2011[41]	40	Poly-herbal Cream		Silver cream		-			-									-	-	-	
Blume 2008[42]	341	NPWT	V.A.C.	Advanced moist wound therapy	+	±			-	+								-	-	-	
Karatepe 2011[43]	67	NPWT	V.A.C.	Standard care	+	+											+	-			
McCallon 2000[44]	10	NPWT	V.A.C.	Saline gauze	-	-												-			
Wang 2011[45]	86	HBOT		EST	→																
Löndahl 2010[46]	94	HBOT		Sham	+					-	-				-			-	-	-	-
Duzgun 2008[47]	100	HBOT		Standard	+					+	+										
Kessler 2003[48]	28	HBOT		Standard	-					-	-								-	-	
Abidia 2003[49]	18	HBOT		Sham	+				-	-	-							-	-	-	
Wainstein 2011[50]	61	Ozone-oxygen	Ozoter	Sham	-	-				-								-			

BD – Biological Dressing; BSE – Biological Skin Equivalent; Col – Collagen; EST – Extracorporeal Shock Wave Therapy; HBOT – Hyperbaric Oxygen Therapy; NaCMC – Sodium Carboxymethylcellulose; NPWT – Negative Pressure Wound Therapy; PDGF – Platelet-derived Growth Factor; PRP – Platelet Rich Plasma

+ Treatment group better than comparator (p< 0.05)
- Treatment group demonstrated no significant benefit
↓ Treatment group worse than comparator
± Significance could not be determined
* + versus std, - versus gel

Table 2. Summary of Baseline Characteristics: Collagen

Characteristic	Number of Studies Reporting	Mean (unless noted)	Range
Number of Patients Randomized	4	489 total	52 - 276
Age (years)	3	57	56 - 59
Gender (% male)	3	74	72 - 77
Race/Ethnicity (%)		-	-
White	2	63	63 - 64
Black	2	10	10 - 12
Other	2	27	25 - 28
Pre-Albumin	1	3.7	-
HbA$_1$C (%)	3	8.4	7.9 - 8.6
Ulcer Size (cm^2)	4	3.1	2.7 - 4.3
Ulcer Duration (months)	4	5.1	3 - 15.1
Infection (%)	4	0	-
Study Duration (weeks)	4	11.3	8 - 12

Secondary Outcomes (Appendix D, Tables 3, 4, and 5)

No difference between Graftjacket and standard care was reported for need for amputation or revascularization surgery.[18] In two studies reporting, there was no significant difference in ulcers infected during treatment between collagen ulcer treatment and standard care.[16,17] Only one study reported the percentage of patients experiencing infection – 12% in the intervention group, 19% in the standard care group.[16] No differences were observed between collagen and standard care in the incidence of adverse events (serious [18% versus 25%] or non-serious [27% versus 25%]),[16] adverse events resulting in study withdrawal (7% overall in one study, 6% versus 0% in a second study, and 6% versus 5% in a third study),[15,17,18] or all-cause mortality (0% in one study, 1.4% versus 4.3% in another study).[16,18]

Biological Dressings

Two studies enrolling 124 patients met eligibility criteria and reported on use of biological dressings in ulcers of diabetic etiology.[19,20] One study described the ulcers as "foot" ulcers; the second study did not provide any information on ulcer location. Both studies were multisite RCTs that took place in the United States; one study also had sites in Canada.[19] One of the trials was of fair quality, industry sponsored, with average ulcer area of 4.1 cm^2 at baseline.[19] The other study was of poor quality, did not include financial disclosures, and had a smaller average baseline ulcer size of 1.9 cm^2.[20] Mean age in the two studies was 59 years and 62% of the enrolled patients were male. Both studies excluded patients with infected ulcers and severe arterial insufficiency. One study reported baseline differences in the distribution of type 1 and type 2 diabetes and the proportion of plantar surface ulcers.[19] One trial included a 1 week run-in period with standard care but did not report if patients were excluded following the run-in period. Compliance with off-loading was monitored in one study.[20] Additional details of the studies are provided in Table 3 and Appendix D, Table 1.

Table 3. Summary of Baseline Characteristics: Biological Dressings

Characteristic	Number of Studies Reporting	Mean (unless noted)	Range
Number of Patients Randomized	2	124 total	26 - 98
Age	2	59	58 - 63
Gender (% male)	2	62	60 - 69
Race/Ethnicity	NR	-	-
BMI	1	33	-
HbA,c (%)	1	8.3	-
ABI	2[a,b]	-	-
Ulcer Size (cm²)	2	3.5	1.9 - 4.1
Ulcer Duration	2[c]		
Study Duration (weeks)	2	12	12

[a]Niezgoda, 2005[19] reported a mean Toe-Brachial-Index (TBI) of 1.00
[b]Mean ABI for Landsman, 2008[20] was not reported, but all participants were >0.65 by exclusion criteria
[c]Landsman 2008:[20] No mean, but >5 weeks duration before treatment per inclusion; Niezgoda 2005:[19] 1-3 months: 49.3%, 4-6 months: 16.4%, 7-12 months: 15.1%, >12 months: 19.2%

Primary Outcomes (Appendix D, Table 2)

Biological dressings were tested against other advanced ulcer care therapies in both studies. One study, a non-inferiority study compared OASIS Wound Matrix biological dressing to rhPDGF [Regranex].[19] For the 73 patients completing the trial, OASIS was no different than rhPDGF for ulcer healing (49% of the OASIS arm and 28% of the Regranex arm had complete ulcer healing at 12 weeks) or time to healing (67 days for OASIS, 73 days for Regranex). The second study compared OASIS to the biological skin equivalent Dermagraft in 26 patients over 12 weeks.[20] No significant difference was noted in complete ulcer healing (77% in OASIS, 85% in Dermagraft) or average time to healing (36 days with OASIS; 41 days with Dermagraft). No comparisons could be made within or between studies regarding the use of ancillary therapies or their effect on healing outcomes.

One study reported on the possible effect of baseline patient characteristics on efficacy, finding in an *a priori* subgroup analysis that the biological dressing did not improve healing of ulcers on the plantar surface compared to rhPDGF. The biological dressing significantly healed more ulcers in patients with type 2 diabetes (p=0.03) but not type 1 diabetes. It is important to note that these subgroup analyses were based on very small sample sizes and only the comparison involving plantar surface ulcers was pre-specified.[19]

Secondary Outcomes (Appendix D, Tables 3, 4, and 5)

Only one study reported any of our secondary outcomes of interest. There were no differences between treatment groups for ulcers infected, ulcer recurrence, pain, proportion of patients experiencing an adverse event, or all-cause mortality.[19]

Biological Skin Equivalents

We identified a total of seven studies that evaluated use of biological skin equivalents in diabetic ulcers; four discussed the use of Dermagraft and three discussed the use of Apligraf. All described the ulcers as "foot" ulcers with no further details on ulcer location. Three fair quality trials with sample sizes of 245,[23] 281,[22] and 50[21] compared Dermagraft (up to 8 grafts) to standard care. A small study (n=26) of poor quality compared Dermagraft (up to 3 grafts) to a biological dressing.[20] All four Dermagraft studies were multisite RCTs that took place in the United States, and all included only ulcers greater than 1.0 cm^2 at baseline (average ulcer size ranged from 1.86 cm^2 to 2.4 cm^2). One study did not report study sponsorship;[20] the others were all industry sponsored. Of the three studies of Apligraf, one was a small trial of poor quality enrolling patients from a single podiatric practice (n=29).[26] Apligraf (up to 5 treatments) was compared to cryopreserved split-thickness skin allograft. This study included ulcers 0.5 to 4.0 cm^2 in size (mean of 1.86 cm^2) and followed patients for 20 weeks. The two other Apligraf trials compared Apligraf to standard care. One enrolled 82 patients in the European Union and Australia[25] and the other enrolled 277 patients in the United States.[24] The trial in Europe and Australia allowed up to 3 treatments over 8 weeks. The trial in the United States allowed up to 5 treatments over 5 weeks. Both were multicenter studies of good quality that included ulcers between 1 and 16 cm^2 in size (average area was approximately 3.0 cm^2) with 12 weeks as the primary endpoint. Overall, 6 of the 7 trials excluded patients with infection and required adequate circulation. The remaining trial did not report on these factors. None of the trials reported on antibiotic use. A run-in period with standard care was included in 4 trials[20,22,24,25] with 2 trials excluding patients whose ulcers decreased in size during the run-in period.[24,25] Five trials reported no differences between treatment groups at baseline; one reported lower age in the control group[21] and one did not report on the groups at baseline.[22] Four of the studies monitored compliance with off-loading either checking the condition of a shoe liner,[20] having patients keep a diary of ambulation,[23] or asking patients about off-loading.[24,25] Additional information is provided in Appendix D, Table 1 and Table 4, below.

Table 4. Summary of Baseline Characteristics: Biological Skin Equivalents

Characteristic	Number of Studies Reporting	Mean (unless noted)	Range
Number of Patients Randomized	7	989 total	26 - 281
Age	5	57	56 - 63
Gender (% male)	5	77	69 - 86
Race/Ethnicity	2[a]		
White	2	71	69 - 72
Other	2	28	28 - 29
BMI	2	32	31 - 32
HbA$_1$c (%)	2	8.6	8.4 - 8.6
ABI	3[b,c]	1	1
Ulcer Size (cm^2)	6	2.6	1.9 - 3.0
Ulcer Duration (weeks)	4	57.1	49.0 - 95.7
Study Duration (weeks)	7	11	8 - 12

[a]Marston, 2003: Caucasian (72%), Non-Caucasian (28%)
Veves, 2001 White (69.5%), African-American (16.6%), Hispanic (13.5%)
[b]Marston, 2003: all participates were >0.7 by exclusion criteria
[c]Veves, 2001: 0.65-0.80: 9.6%, 0.80-1.00: 33.2%, >1.0: 54.4%

Primary Outcomes (Appendix D, Table 2)

Three studies compared Dermagraft to standard care. Two of these showed statistically significant improvements in ulcer healing. One reported that Dermagraft resulted in an increased incidence of complete ulcer healing (30.0% versus 18.3%, p=0.049) and resulted in a faster time to closure (p=0.04).[23] The second study also found a benefit in the proportion of completely healed ulcers with weekly Dermagraft administration (50% versus 8%, Fisher's exact test p=0.03). A statistical benefit in time to closure was not reached (p=0.056) due to small group sizes.[21] The third trial comparing Dermagraft to standard care did not show a benefit for the treatment group when taken as a whole.[22] However, among patients who received a metabolically active Dermagraft at least for the first implant, the percentage of ulcers healed was significantly higher than those who received standard care (49% versus 32%, p<0.01).[22] In this older trial, some of the Dermagraft samples were found to have a level of metabolic activity outside of the therapeutic range. We pooled the findings from the three studies of Dermagraft versus standard care (Figure 2). The overall risk ratio was 1.49 (95% CI 0.96 to 2.32) indicating a non-significant benefit of Dermagraft over standard care in ulcer healing. The fourth study compared Dermagraft (up to 3 applications) to the biological dressing OASIS in 26 patients and, as noted above, found both produced similar improvements for incidence and time to complete ulcer healing.[20]

Figure 2. Proportion of Diabetic Ulcers Healed - Biological Skin Equivalent (Dermagraft) versus Standard Care

Study or Subgroup	Control Events	Total	Treatment Events	Total	Weight	Risk Ratio M-H, Random, 95% CI	Risk Ratio M-H, Random, 95% CI
Gentzkow 1996	6	12	1	13	4.7%	6.50 [0.91, 46.43]	
Marston 2003	39	130	21	115	42.1%	1.64 [1.03, 2.62]	
Naughton 1997	42	109	40	126	53.2%	1.21 [0.86, 1.72]	
Total (95% CI)		**251**		**254**	**100.0%**	**1.49 [0.96, 2.32]**	
Total events	87		62				

Heterogeneity: Tau² = 0.06; Chi² = 3.53, df = 2 (P = 0.17); I² = 43%
Test for overall effect: Z = 1.78 (P = 0.08)

0.2 0.5 1 2 5
Favors Control   Favors Dermagraft

*Gentzkow 1996 – Analysis is for Group A (one piece of Dermagraft applied weekly) versus Control

The two largest studies of Apligraf used standard care (sharp debridement, moist dressings, and off-loading) as the comparator. The largest study[24] showed significant benefit for Apligraf in complete ulcer healing at 12 weeks (56% versus 38%, p=0.004) and for median time to closure (65 versus 90 days for control, p=0.003). The second trial[25] also showed a significant benefit for Apligraf for incidence of complete ulcer healing (52% versus 26%, p=0.049), but the benefit of more rapid healing did not reach statistical significance (p=0.059) before trial enrollment was prematurely terminated due to registration difficulties. Pooled analysis of these trials (Figure 3) shows a significant overall benefit of Apligraf over standard care (ARD=21%, 95% CI 9% to 32%; RR=1.58, 95% CI 1.20 to 2.08, I²=0%). The third study compared Apligraf to cryopreserved split-thickness skin allografts. This small (n=29 ulcers), poor-quality study did not report statistically significant differences between treatments for the incidence of complete ulcer healing or time to complete healing.[26]

Figure 3. Proportion of Diabetic Ulcers Healed - Biological Skin Equivalent (Apligraf) versus Standard Care

Study or Subgroup	Apligraf Events	Total	Standard Care Events	Total	Weight	Risk Ratio M-H, Random, 95% CI	Risk Ratio M-H, Random, 95% CI
Edmonds 2009	17	33	10	38	19.2%	1.96 [1.05, 3.66]	
Veves 2001	63	112	36	96	80.8%	1.50 [1.11, 2.04]	
Total (95% CI)		145		134	100.0%	1.58 [1.20, 2.08]	
Total events	80		46				

Heterogeneity: Tau² = 0.00; Chi² = 0.56, df = 1 (P = 0.45); I² = 0%
Test for overall effect: Z = 3.26 (P = 0.001)

0.2   0.5   1   2   5
Favors Std Care   Favors Apligraf

No comparisons could be made within or between studies regarding the use of ancillary therapies. However, in one study, were allowed to be ambulatory, using extra-depth custom inserts or healing sandals.[23] Patients recorded being on their feet an average of 8 hours a day. Most other studies limited patients to use of a wheelchair or crutches for large portions of the study or asked patients to limit ambulation to a minimal level. While no controlled comparisons can be made, it is important to note that use of Dermagraft in this trial still produced a beneficial effect. This suggests the benefits of this biological skin equivalent may be maintained when applied to clinic patients not willing or able to limit ambulation for several months during the period of treatment.

Two of the Dermagraft studies reported on factors associated with ulcer healing. In one study, neither patient age, gender, ulcer size or duration, diabetes type, ankle-arm index, nor HbA$_1$c were significantly associated with time to closure.[21] Another study reported outcomes based on ulcer location.[23] There was a trend for more forefoot/toe ulcers (n=214) to heal with Dermagraft (29.5% versus 19.6%, p=0.065). For heel ulcers (n=31), 33% of those treated with Dermagraft achieved closure compared to 8% in the control group (p=0.01). This trial was originally intended to include ulcers of any duration. At interim analysis, the benefits of Dermagraft on ulcer healing were not statistically significant when considering all patients, but a statistically significant benefit was evident for the treatment of ulcers present for more than 6 weeks prior to entering the 2 week screening. This resulted in a trial amendment to change the desired study population and further enroll only chronic ulcers of more than 6 weeks.

Secondary Outcomes (Appendix D, Tables 3, 4, and 5)

Rate of recurrence was reported for two of the Dermagraft studies with no difference between the Dermagraft and standard care groups.[21,22] Similarly, two studies reported no significant difference in rate of recurrence between Apligraf and standard care.[24,25] Three Dermagraft studies[22-23] and one Apligraf study[25] reported no differences between a biological skin equivalent and standard care in incidence of ulcers infected during treatment. One Dermagraft study found a significantly lower incidence of infection, osteomyelitis, and cellulitus (combined) in the Dermagraft group than in the standard care group (19% versus 33%, p=0.007).[23] One Apligraf study found a significantly lower incidence of osteomyelitis (but not infection or cellulitis) in the advanced therapy group compared to standard care (2.7% versus 10.4%, p=0.04).[24] One study reported fewer amputations among patients treated with Apligraf than standard care (6% versus 16%, p=0.03)[24] although a second study found no significant difference.[25] No studies reported pain or discomfort. Six studies reported a low number of patients experiencing adverse events, adverse events leading to study withdrawal, or all-cause mortality with no differences between the biological skin equivalent and either standard care[21-25] or allograft.[26]

Platelet-Derived Wound Healing (Platelet-Derived Growth Factors, PDGF)

Nine randomized controlled trials enrolling a total of 990 patients evaluated the efficacy of platelet-derived growth factors (PDGFs) used in the treatment of diabetic ulcers. Comparator treatments included standard care or placebo,[28-34] biological dressing,[19] silver sulfadiazine,[27] and either standard care or sodium carboxymethylcellulose (NaCMC) gel.[35] Ulcer locations were described as lower limb or lower extremity in 5 studies,[29,31-35] foot in 2 studies,[28,30] with one specifying plantar surface,[30] and not defined in 2 studies.[19,27] Four studies were conducted in India,[28-30,32] three in the United States,[31,33-35] one in the United States and Canada,[19] and one in Iran.[27] Five of nine studies reported a funding source; four received industry funding[19,31,33-35] and one reported government support.[27] The mean age of the participants was 58 years; 69 percent were males (Table 5). PDGF trials ranged in duration from eight to twenty weeks and all included chronic, non-healing, diabetic ulcers of at least four weeks in duration. Three studies excluded patients with infection and the remaining studies required infection to be controlled before starting the study therapy. Six trials allowed antibiotics during the study on an as needed basis. Eight studies reported only including patients with adequate blood flow; one provided no information on blood supply. Three studies reported monitoring compliance with care. One tracked dressing changes and off-loading,[29] one provided a diary to record dressing changes,[33,34] and the third reported compliance but did not specify what was monitored.[31] Two studies included a run-in period.[27,29] Inclusion criteria across studies allowed for ulcer sizes ranging from 1 cm^2 to 100 cm^2; average ulcer size was 7.3 cm^2. One study reported a significant difference in ulcer area at baseline with larger ulcers found in the PDGF arm (54.3 cm^2 versus 28.7 cm^2 in the control arm, p=0.003).[28] As noted in the section on biological dressings (above) one trial reported baseline differences in ulcer location (plantar vs. non-plantar) and distribution of type 1 and type 2 diabetes between groups.[19] No trials reported a difference between treatments in ulcer duration or use of ancillary therapies. Two studies were good quality,[32-34] 5 were fair quality,[19,28,30,31,35] and 2 were poor quality.[27,29] A complete summary of study characteristics is presented in Appendix D, Table 1.

Table 5. Summary of Baseline Characteristics: Platelet-Derived Growth Factor

Characteristic	Number of Studies Reporting	Mean (unless noted)	Range
Number of Patients Randomized	9	990 total	9 - 382
Age (years)	9	58	51 - 61
Gender (% male)	8	69	60 - 100
Race/Ethnicity (%)			
White	3	83	81 - 86
Black	2	11	9.9 - 12
Hispanic	1	6	-
Asian	1	<1	-
Indian	1	100	-
Other	3	4	0.3 - 14
BMI	4	27.4	22.4 - 32.5

HbA$_1$c (%)	3	8.0	7.5 - 8.8
ABI	2	1.1	1.1
Ulcer Size (cm²)	9	7.3	2.7 - 41.5
Ulcer Duration (weeks)	5[a]	48	13 - 78[a]
Infection	4	0	-
Study Duration (weeks)	9	16	8 - 20
History of Amputation	2[b]	35	-
History of PVD	1	0	-

[a]Jaiswal 2010[32] reported a median of 5 weeks
[b]Jaiswal 2010[32] reported amputation or previous ulcer (2%) and was not included in the calculation

Primary Outcomes (Appendix D, Table 2)

All nine trials reported the percentage of ulcers healed by study completion for PDGF and comparator. Seven of nine compared PDGF to placebo or inactive gel[28,29,31-34] or to standard ulcer care[30,35] and three of nine compared PDGF to another advanced wound therapy.[19,27,35] A pooled analysis of the studies comparing PDGF to placebo gel or standard ulcer care (Figure 4) found significantly greater healing with PDGF (ARD=21%, 95% CI 14% to 29%; RR=1.45, 95% CI 1.03 to 2.05) but there was substantial heterogeneity (I^2=85%). Five of the seven individual trials also showed significantly greater healing with PDGF with individual risk ratios ranging from 1.60 to 3.00.

Separate analyses of studies with placebo gel and standard care as comparators revealed a significant finding for the 5 placebo gel studies (RR=1.45, 95% CI 1.07 to 1.97, I^2=63%) and a non-significant finding for the 2 standard care studies (RR=1.40, 95% CI 0.33 to 5.95, I^2=96%). Pooling only studies rated as good or fair quality showed no benefit of PDGF compared to placebo gel or standard care (RR=1.45, 95% CI 0.94 to 2.23) with substantial heterogeneity (I^2=80%). An analysis based on the country in which the study was conducted found a significant benefit of PDGF over placebo gel in 2 studies done in the United States (RR=1.54, 95% CI 1.19 to 2.00, I^2=0%) but not in 3 studies done in India (RR=1.39, 95% CI 0.77 to 2.51, I^2=79%). Significant results favoring PDGF were also found for studies with more than 100 patients (k=3), but not studies with less than 100 (k=2) and studies with treatment lasting 20 weeks (k=3) but not studies less than 20 weeks (k=3 due to multiple reporting times in one trial). Ulcer size did not appear to be a factor with non-significant findings when pooling the 2 studies with the largest ulcer sizes (greater than 25 cm²) or the 3 studies with ulcer size less than 25 cm².

Three of nine studies reported the percentage of ulcers healed by study completion for PDGF compared to another advanced wound therapy. The percentage of ulcers healed did not differ significantly for PDGF compared to biological dressings (OASIS),[19] silver sulfadiazine,[27] or NaCMC gel[35] (Figure 4).

Figure 4. Proportion of Diabetic Ulcers Healed – Platelet-Derived Growth Factor versus Comparator

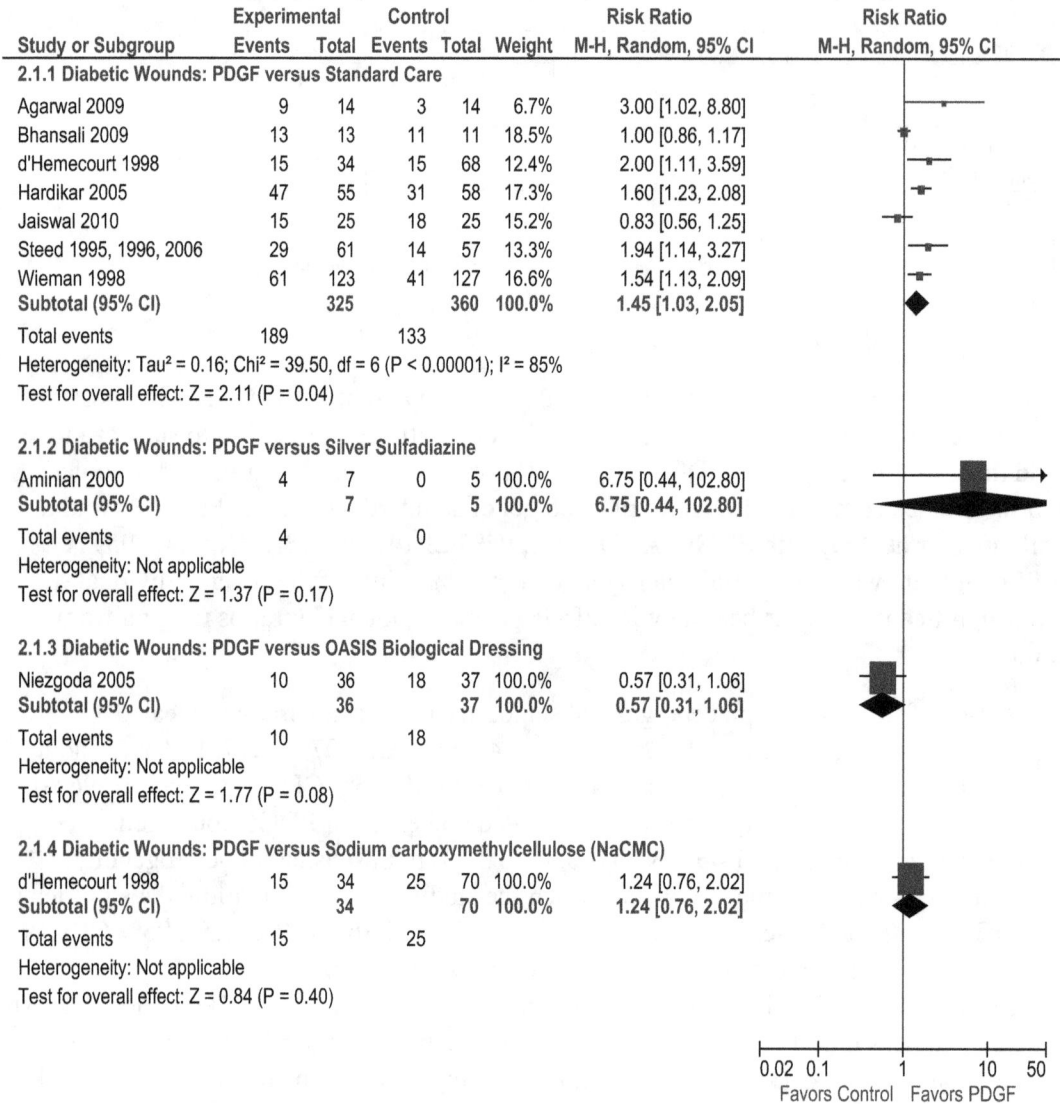

Five studies reported time to complete ulcer closure for PDGF compared to placebo gel or standard care.[29-31,33-35] Four of the five studies reported significantly shorter time to ulcer healing in PDGF compared to placebo gel or standard care (differences of 30 to 40 days);[29-31,33,34] one study found no significant difference.[35] In studies comparing PDGF to another advanced therapy, time to complete ulcer closure did not differ significantly for PDGF compared to biological dressings (OASIS),[19] silver sulfadiazine,[27] or NaCMC gel.[35]

Several individual studies looked at factors associated with ulcer healing. In one study, ulcers less than 9 cm², ulcers located on non-weight-bearing surfaces, and the use of antibiotics significantly improved healing.[29] Another study reported that healing did not vary by age and baseline HbA_1c but that compliance with off-loading was positively associated with healing (p not reported).[31] As noted above, healing of plantar surface ulcers was comparable for patients treated with either a biological dressing or rhPDGF.[19]

Secondary Outcomes (Appendix D, Tables 3, 4, and 5)

Four studies reported the percentage of ulcers infected during treatment with no significant differences between PDGF and placebo or standard care,[31,33-35] a biological dressing,[19] or NaCMC gel.[35] Three studies reported ulcer recurrence with no significant differences between PDGF and placebo or standard care[31,33,34] or a biological dressing.[19] Time to recurrence was similar between PDGF and placebo in the one study reporting that outcome.[33,34] Pain or discomfort was reported in four studies with no significant differences between PDGF and placebo or standard care,[31,33-35] a biological dressing,[19] or NaCMC gel.[35] Three studies found no significant difference between PDGF and placebo gel or standard care[29,31,35] or between PDGF and NaCMC gel[35] for patient withdrawals attributed to adverse events. Two studies reported no adverse events during the study period[30,32] and three studies found no significant difference in the occurrence of adverse events between treatment groups (PDGF versus placebo gel,[33,34] standard care,[35] biological dressing,[19] or NaCMC.[35] All-cause mortality was reported in five studies with no significant difference between PDGF and standard care, placebo, or other advanced treatments.[19,29,31,33-35] Only one study reported allergic reaction to the treatment with no difference between PDGF and placebo gel.[28]

Platelet Rich Plasma (PRP)

Two randomized controlled trials met eligibility criteria and compared the efficacy of PRP to placebo gel[37] or platelet poor plasma (PPP).[36] One study was conducted in the United States and reported government funding[37] and one was done in Egypt with no funding source reported.[36] Study quality was rated as poor for one trial[36] and fair for the second.[37] Ulcer location was described only as "foot" for one study;[36] the other study included plantar, medial, and lateral ulcers (including 38% on the toes and 29% on the heel).[37] One study reported patient age (57 years) and gender (80% male).[37] The trial durations were twelve[37] or twenty weeks,[36] and included chronic, non-healing ulcers greater than four[37] or twelve[36] weeks in duration. Treatments were applied two times a week with 3 to 4 day intervals between dressing changes until the respective study duration was complete or healing had occurred. Both studies excluded patients with infection and inadequate blood flow. Antibiotic use was not reported nor was compliance with treatment. One study reported no baseline differences between groups;[36] the second reported differences in race in the per protocol analysis sample.[37] One study included a 1-week run-in period and excluded patients if ulcer area decreased by more than 50%.[37] Inclusion criteria allowed for all ulcers greater than 0.5 cm²; the average enrolled ulcer size was 5.6 cm². Neither trial reported a difference between treatment arms in ulcer size, ulcer duration, or ancillary therapies. Additional baseline characteristics are presented in Table 6. A complete summary of study characteristics is presented in Appendix D, Table 1.

Table 6. Summary of Baseline Characteristics: Platelet Rich Plasma

Characteristic	Number of Studies Reporting	Mean (unless noted)	Range
Number of Patients Randomized	2	96 total	24 - 72
Age (years)	1	57	-
Gender (% male)	1	80	-
Race/Ethnicity (%)			
White	1	60	-
Black	1	7.5	-
Hispanic	1	30	-
Other	1	2.5	-
HbA,c (%)	1	7.9	-
Smoking	1	33.3	-
Ulcer Size (cm^2)	2	5.6	3.5 - 9.4
Infection	1	0	-
Study Duration (weeks)	2	11	12 - 20
History of HTN (%)	1	70	-

Primary Outcomes (Appendix D, Table 2)

Both trials reported the percentage of ulcers healed by study completion for PRP compared to PPP (100% versus 75%)[36] or placebo gel (33% versus 28%).[37] Neither difference was significant. One study[36] reported a significantly shorter time to healed ulcers for PRP compared to PPP (11.5 versus 17 weeks, p<0.005); the other study found no significant difference between treatment groups.[37]

Secondary Outcomes (Appendix D, Tables 3, 4, and 5)

One study reported no difference in ulcer recurrence at 12 weeks between PRP and placebo gel.[37] This trial also reported no significant differences in adverse events or all-cause mortality.[37] The second study did not report any secondary outcomes.

Silver Products

Four trials enrolling a total of 280 patients met eligibility criteria.[38-41] One study compared silver ointment to standard care[38] and one compared a silver dressing to a calcium-based dressing.[40] In two trials, silver cream was the control group; the interventions were oak bark extract[39] and a polyherbal treatment.[41] The studies were done in the United States,[39] Europe,[40] Italy,[38] and India.[41] Two reported industry support[40,41] and two did not report a funding source. Enrollments ranged from 40[39,41] to 134.[40] Ulcer locations were described as "foot" for two studies[38,40] with one specifying that 68% were plantar and 32% were non-plantar.[40] The other two studies included only plantar surface ulcers.[39,41] One study excluded patients with infection (with antibiotic use during the trial not reported),[39] one study excluded patients with "severe" infection and allowed antibiotic use during the trial,[41] one study stratified patients based on antibiotic use,[40] and one noted that infection was the cause of some of the included ulcers (antibiotic use not reported).[38] Three studied required adequate blood supply;[38-40] the fourth allowed patients with peripheral arterial disease.[41] None of the studies included a run-in period with standard care, none reported monitoring compliance with therapy, two specified off-loading as part of standard care, and none reported baseline differences between treatment groups. All studies were of fair quality. Study characteristics are summarized in Table 7; more detail is provided in Appendix D, Table 1.

Table 7. Summary of Baseline Characteristics: Silver Products

Characteristic	Number of Studies Reporting	Mean (unless noted)	Range
Number of Patients Randomized	4	280 total	40 - 134
Age (years)	3	58.7	55.9 - 60.0
Gender (% male)	2	58.6	44 - 74
Race/Ethnicity (%)	NR		
HbA$_1$c (%)	2	8.6	8.0 - 10.7
ABI	1	1.8	-
Ulcer Size (cm^2)	2[a]	3.2	2.2 - 3.7
Ulcer Duration (months)	2	12.3	0.48 - 15.6
Infection (%)	1[b]	100	-
Study Duration (weeks)	3	6.6	4 - 8
History of PVD	1	23.7%	-

[a]One study included only ulcers ≤3 cm in diameter; one study reported mean length of 4.6 cm and mean width of 3.3 cm
[b]Three studies excluded patients with clinical signs of infection or taking antibiotics at screening

One study included only ulcers with a diameter of 3 cm or less.[39] In the other studies, the mean ulcer size was 2.2 cm^2,[38] 3.7 cm^2,[40] or 4.6 cm (length) and 3.3 cm (width).[41] Mean ulcer duration was 14.5 days in one study[41] and 1.3 years in another.[40] Two studies did not report duration. Two studies included only Wagner Grade 1 or 2 ulcers[39,40] while a third included Grade 1, 2, or 3 ulcers.[41]

Three studies were done to assess the efficacy and safety of the intervention for ulcer healing.[38,40,41] The fourth study was focused on reduction in size of the ulcer.[39]

Primary Outcomes (Appendix D, Table 2)

Three of the four studies reported percentage of ulcers healed. In one study, the percentage of ulcers healed at 4 weeks was significantly higher in the group treated with silver ointment than the group receiving standard care (39% versus 16%, ARD=23%, 95% CI 2% to 43%, p<0.05). Mean size of the ulcers included in the study was 2.2 cm^2.[38] Mean time to healing was not reported. In two other studies that reported healing, one found no difference in healed ulcers after 6 weeks of treatment, between an oak bark extract and a silver cream (40% versus 30%, respectively).[39] The second study found no difference in healed ulcers (31% versus 22%) or time to healing (53 days versus 58 days) for a silver dressing compared to a calcium dressing.[40] The findings for proportion of ulcers healed are presented in Figure 5. The study comparing silver and calcium dressings also reported a global assessment of healing with 88% of ulcers healed or improved in the silver dressing group compared to 71% in the calcium dressing group (a non-significant difference).[40] Subgroup analyses based on location (plantar, non-plantar) and type of ulcer (neuropathic, neuroischemic) also were non-significant. The only significant finding was a greater percentage of ulcers healed or improved (92% versus 50%) in the silver dressing group among patients taking systemic antibiotics at baseline.[40] The third study reported only time to healing with no difference between a polyherbal extract and a silver cream (43 days versus 44 days).[41]

Figure 5. Proportion of Diabetic Ulcers Healed – Silver Products

Study or Subgroup	Silver Events	Total	Control Events	Total	Risk Ratio M-H, Random, 95% CI	Risk Ratio M-H, Random, 95% CI
1.1.1 Silver cream versus standard care						
Belcaro 2010	13	34	5	32	2.45 [0.98, 6.09]	
1.1.2 Silver cream versus oak bark extract						
Jacobs 2008	6	20	8	20	0.75 [0.32, 1.77]	
1.1.3 Silver dressing versus calcium dressing						
Jude 2008	21	67	15	67	1.40 [0.79, 2.47]	

0.1 0.2 0.5 1 2 5 10
Favors Control   Favors Silver

Secondary Outcomes (Appendix D, Tables 3, 4, and 5)

Few secondary outcomes were reported. Two studies found no difference in ulcers infected during treatment when a silver dressing was compared to a calcium dressing[40] or a silver cream was compared to a polyherbal cream.[41] There was also no difference in ulcer recurrence between a silver cream and a polyherbal cream (42% versus 47%, respectively).[41] Adverse events and withdrawals from the study due to adverse events were comparable for the two treatment groups within each of the four studies. In three studies, no patients experienced adverse events.[38,39,41] In the fourth study, 37% of patients in the silver dressing group experienced an adverse event compared to 39% of those in the calcium dressing group.[40] Serious adverse events were reported in 12% and 16% of participants, respectively, with study-related adverse events in 16% and 13%, respectively.[40] All-cause mortality was reported in two studies. Overall values were low (maximum of 1 patient per group) with no differences between a silver dressing and a calcium dressing[40] or a silver cream and a polyherbal cream.[41] Two studies assessed allergic reactions to treatments but reported no events.[38,39]

Negative Pressure Wound Therapy

Three trials of NPWT met inclusion criteria. In one study, a small pilot study with 10 patients, the goal of NPWT was to prepare the ulcer for final closure.[44] In the other two studies, with enrollments of 341[42] and 67[43] the goal was ulcer healing. All three studies compared NPWT to standard care. Ulcer location was described as "foot" for two studies[43,44] and calcaneal, dorsal, or plantar for the third study.[42] Two studies were done in the United States[42,44] and one in Turkey.[43] One study received industry support[42] while no source of funding was reported for the other two studies.[43,44] One study was of good quality.[42] Quality of the other two studies could not accurately be assessed due to either incomplete reporting[43] or the fact that the study was a small pilot study.[44] Study characteristics are presented in Table 8 and Appendix D, Table 1.

Table 8. Summary of Baseline Characteristics: Negative Pressure Wound Therapy

Characteristic	Number of Studies Reporting	Mean (unless noted)	Range
Number of Patients Randomized	3	418 total	10 - 341
Age (years)	3	60	53 - 67
Gender (% male)	2	70	28 - 78
Race/Ethnicity (%)			
White	1	58	-
Black	1	15	-
Hispanic	1	24	-
Native American	1	2	-
Other	1	1	-
Pre-Albumin	1	20.5	-
HbA$_1$c (%)	1	8.2	-
Smoking	1	19	-
ABI	1	1.0	-
Ulcer Size (cm^2)	2	15.7	12.3 - 32.4
Ulcer Duration (weeks)	2	26	10 - 29
Study Duration (weeks)	2 [a]	10	8 - 12

[a]One study followed participants to healing (mean of 4 months)

The mean age of study participants was 60 years. Two studies reported gender with 78%[42] and 28%[43] male. Only one study reported race with 58% Caucasian, 24% Hispanic, and 15% African-American.[42] Initial ulcer sizes and ulcer durations were reported in the two studies with complete healing as the goal. Mean size (duration) was 12.3 cm^2 (29 weeks) in one study[42] and 32.4 cm^2 (10 weeks) in the other.[43] No study reported on comorbid conditions other than diabetes. Two studies reported excluding patients with either venous disease[44] or inadequate lower extremity perfusion.[42] These studies also excluded patients with active or uncontrolled infection. Antibiotic use during the trial was not reported but both reported that off-loading was a component of care for all[44] or 97.5%[42] of patients. One study reported excluding patients for non-compliance but did not specify how that was determined.[42] None of the trials required a run-in period with standard care and two reported no baseline differences between groups.[42,43]

Primary Outcomes (Appendix D, Table 2)

Percentage of ulcers healed was reported in only one of the trials.[42] In that trial, 43% of the patients treated with NPWT experienced ulcer healing compared to 29% of those treated with standard care (ARD=14%, 95% CI 4% to 24%, p<0.05). Median time to ulcer healing was 96 days (13.7 weeks) in the NPWT group but could not be estimated in the standard care group. In the second trial with complete healing as the goal, mean time to healing was reported to be significantly shorter (4.2 versus 5.3 weeks, p<0.05) among patients receiving NPWT compared to those receiving standard care.[43] The third trial reported satisfactory healing (definitive closure of the ulcer) at a mean of 3.3 weeks in the NPWT group and at a mean of 6.1 weeks in the standard care group; the difference was not significant.[44] In the NPWT group, 80% (4 of 5) ulcers achieved complete closure by delayed primary intention (skin graft, myocutaneous flap, or suture closure by surgeon) compared to 40% (2 of 5) in the standard care group. We pooled time to complete healing data from these two studies (Figure 6) and found a significant benefit for patients treated with NPWT (mean difference=-8.07, 95% CI -13.70 to -2.45, p=0.005).

Figure 6. Time to Complete Healing, Diabetic Ulcers – Negative Pressure Wound Therapy

Study or Subgroup	NPWT Mean	SD	Total	Control Mean	SD	Total	Weight	Mean Difference IV, Random, 95% CI	Mean Difference IV, Random, 95% CI
Karatepe 2011	29.4	13.3	30	37.1	9.8	37	97.0%	-7.70 [-13.41, -1.99]	
McCallon 2000	22.8	17.4	5	42.8	32.5	5	3.0%	-20.00 [-52.31, 12.31]	
Total (95% CI)			**35**			**42**	**100.0%**	**-8.07 [-13.70, -2.45]**	

Heterogeneity: Tau² = 0.00; Chi² = 0.54, df = 1 (P = 0.46); I² = 0%
Test for overall effect: Z = 2.81 (P = 0.005)

-100   -50   0   50   100
Favors NPWT   Favors Control

Secondary Outcomes (Appendix D, Tables 3, 4, and 5)

In one study, although more ulcers became infected during NPWT (2.4% versus 0.6% in the standard care group, p=ns), significantly fewer patients in the NPWT group required a secondary amputation (4.1% versus 10.2%, p<0.05).[42] One study reported a positive effect of NPTW on the mental (p=0.03) and physical (p=0.004) health components of the SF-36 compared to conventional treatment.[43] Two studies reported no significant differences in withdrawals due to adverse events or all-cause mortality.[42,44]

Hyperbaric Oxygen Therapy (HBOT)

HBOT versus Standard Care With or Without Sham

Four RCTs evaluating adjunctive hyperbaric oxygen therapy (HBOT) for the treatment of chronic diabetic ulcers met inclusion criteria (Table 9).[46-49] One of the trials enrolled patients with ischemic diabetic ulcers.[49] Ulcers were described as located on the lower extremity,[49] below the ankle,[46] and "foot".[47] One study reported that 61% of the ulcers were on the heel or sole and 39% were on the toe.[48] A total of 240 patients, 123 receiving HBOT and 117 receiving control, with a mean age of 65 were enrolled. Most patients were male (57%). Comorbidities were not uniformly reported but some of the trials reported histories of coronary or cardiovascular disease, hypertension, or hyperlipidemia (see Appendix D, Table 1). The trials were conducted in Europe[46,48,49] or Turkey.[47]

Table 9. Summary of Baseline Characteristic: Hyperbaric Oxygen Therapy versus Standard Care/Sham

Characteristic	Number of Studies Reporting	Mean (unless noted)	Range
Number of Patients Randomized	4	244 total	18 - 100
Age (years)	4	65	61 - 71
Gender (% male)	4	57	32 - 81
Race/Ethnicity (%)	NR		
HbA₁c (%)	3	8.2	7.9 - 8.8
Smoking	3	39	19 - 56
History of CAD/CVD (%)	2	27	22 - 29
History of Amputation (%)	3	36	11 - 39
History of HTN (%)	2	67	60 - 75
Wagner Wound Grade I (%)	1*	6	-
Wagner Wound Grade II (%)	3*	28	18 - 94
Wagner Wound Grade III (%)	3*	42	0 - 56
Wagner Wound Grade IV (%)	3*	29	0 - 45
Treatment Duration (weeks)	4	2 - 8	
Follow-up Duration (weeks)	4	2 - 92	

*One trial reported I through III with no further detail

Inclusion varied by ulcer grade, size, and duration (Table 10). Based on Wagner classification, 28% were wound grade 2 (range 18 to 94), 42% wound grade 3 (range 0 to 56), and 29% ulcer grade 4 (range 0 to 45).[46,47,49] One trial reported Wagner grades 1-3 with no further details.[48] Mean ulcer sizes at baseline were 2.6 cm$^{2(48)}$ and 3.0 cm^2.[46] One trial specified ulcer size between >1 cm between <10 cm.[49] Duration of ulcers required for inclusion ranged from at least 4 weeks to at least 3 months. Two studies allowed patients with infected ulcers to enroll,[47,49] one study enrolled patients when the infection was controlled,[46] and the third excluded patients with severe sepsis.[48] All trials allowed antibiotics, as needed. One study enrolled patients with ischemic ulcers,[49] two studies excluded patients with ischemia,[46,48] and one did not report exclusion criteria related to ischemia.[47] In three of the studies, the patients had to have completed at least 6 weeks of standard care.[46,48,49] These trials also specified off-loading as part of standard care. One study excluded patients for suspected poor compliance,[46] one noted that the protocol was followed,[49] one hospitalized patients for 2 weeks,[48] and one did not report on compliance.[47] There were variations between trials on the applications of HBOT. Treatment pressure (atmospheres absolute) ranged from 2 to 3 ATA, typically around 2.5 ATA. Treatment periods ranged from 2 weeks[48] to 8 weeks[46] with the number of sessions ranging from 20 to approximately 40. One session was 90 minutes. The control arms utilized standard multi-disciplinary ulcer care but two of the trials also used an adjunct blinded sham procedure.[46,49] Mean follow-up times ranged from 2 weeks[48] to 92 weeks.[47]

The aggregate study quality of the included trials was fair. Only one study satisfactorily met the four study quality domains.[49] In one study, there were statistically significant differences at baseline in the percentage of males, current smokers, obese patients, all more prevalent in the HBOT arm.[47]

Table 10. Ulcer Size, Ulcer Duration, and Definitions of Closure: Hyperbaric Oxygen Therapy versus Standard Care/Sham

Study / Location	Mean ulcer size, cm² (range or SD)	Duration of ulcer, months (range)	Definition of ulcer closure
Löndahl 2010 / Sweden[46]	HBOT: 3.1 (0.6 to 55) Control: 2.8 (0.6 to 55)	HBOT: 9 (3 to 44) Control: 10 (3 to 39)	Complete epithelial regeneration and remaining so until the next visit in the study
Duzgun 2008 / Turkey[47]	HBOT: NR Control: NR	HBOT: NR Control: NR	Total closure of the ulcer without the need for surgical intervention in the operating room
Abidia 2003 / UK[49]	HBOT: 10.6 (1.2 to 82.3) Control: 7.8 (1.8 to 86.6)	HBOT: 6 (2 to 18) Control: 9 (3 to 60)	Complete epithelialization
Kessler 2003 / France[48]	HBOT: 2.31 (2.18) Control: 2.82 (2.43)	HBOT: NR, ≥3 mos Control: NR, ≥3 mos	Not reported

Primary Outcomes (Appendix D, Table 2)

Due to variations in follow-up durations all of the trials could not be statistically pooled (Figure 7). Three of the trials had a follow-up duration of at least one year[46,47,49] and one trial evaluated ulcer healing within 2 weeks of therapy.[48] One long-term, placebo-controlled trial (1-year of follow-up) reported that 52% of patients allocated to adjunctive HBOT had completely healed ulcers compared to 29% of patients in the control arm (RR=1.85, 95% CI 1.05 to 3.16).[46] Another smaller sham-controlled trial (n=18) found a higher proportion of patients[49] with healed ischemic diabetic ulcers with adjunct HBOT compared to control at one year, 63% versus 0% (p=0.026, Fisher's exact test), respectively. Another long-term study (n=100) with a mean follow-up duration of 92 weeks reported that 66% of patients receiving adjunct HBOT had completely healed ulcers without requiring surgery versus 0% of the patients in the standard therapy arm ($p<0.001$).[47] In the short-term trial by Kessler, within 2 weeks of therapy 2 of 14 patients had complete healing versus none of the 13 patients in the control group.[48] None of the studies reported mean time to healing.

Figure 7. Proportion of Diabetic Ulcers Healed – Hyperbaric Oxygen Therapy

Study or Subgroup	HBOT Events	HBOT Total	Control Events	Control Total	Risk Ratio M-H, Random, 95% CI
1.2.1 HBOT versus sham (+ multidisicplinary wound care, both arms): any duration					
Abidia 2003	5	8	0	8	11.00 [0.71, 170.98]
Duzgun 2008	33	50	0	50	67.00 [4.22, 1064.23]
Kessler 2003	2	14	0	13	4.67 [0.24, 88.96]
Londahl 2010	25	48	12	42	1.82 [1.05, 3.16]
1.2.5 HBOT versus Extracorporeal shockwave therapy: short-term duration (4 weeks)					
Wang 2011	10	40	24	44	0.46 [0.25, 0.84]

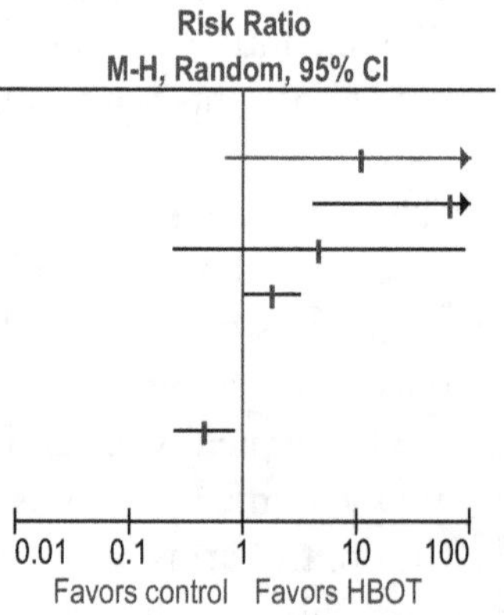

Secondary Outcomes (Appendix D, Tables 3, 4, and 5)

In one study, four major amputations and eight minor amputations were performed within the first year but differences between the HBOT and sham treatment groups were not significant.[46] A second study also reported no differences between HBOT and sham treatment in major or minor amputations.[49] One study, however, did report fewer distal and proximal amputations and fewer debridement procedures in the HBOT group than in the standard therapy group.[47] All of the standard therapy patients required some form of surgical management (i.e. debridement, graft or flap, or distal amputation) to achieve ulcer closure compared to 8 (16%) patients in the HBOT group.[47]

Other reported secondary outcomes included no difference between HBOT and sham treatment in the number of percutaneous transluminal angioplasty procedures done[46] and no difference between HBOT and sham treatment in ulcers infected during treatment.[49]

Adverse events, reported in 2 studies,[48,49] and withdrawals due to adverse events, reported in all 4 studies.[46-49] did not differ between HBOT and sham treatment or standard care. Three trials reported all-cause mortality with no deaths in 2 studies[48,49] and a non-significant difference between HBOT and sham treatment in the third.[46] Two studies observed barometric otitis in one patient in the HBOT group and no patients in the sham treatment or standard care groups.[46,48] No incidences of oxygen toxicity were reported.

HBOT versus Extracorporeal Shockwave Therapy

One comparative effectiveness study conducted in Taiwan compared HBOT (38 patients/40 feet) to extracorporeal shockwave therapy (EST, 39 patients/44 feet).[45] Mean age of the patients was 62 years; gender was not reported. Median size of the ulcers was 7 cm^2 (range 2 to 12) in the HBOT group and 4 cm^2 (range 1.5 to 9) in the EST group, a nearly statistically significant difference (p=0.059). Median duration of the ulcers was 6 months. Patients with active infection were excluded but could be enrolled when no sepsis or necrosis. Antibiotics were used as needed during the trial. There were no inclusion or exclusion criteria related to blood supply and no run-in with standard care. HBOT was performed in a sealed multi-place chamber at a pressure of 2.5 ATA five times per week for a total of 20 treatments over four weeks duration. EST was performed with a dermaPACE device (Sanuwave, Alpharetta, GA). Treatment dosage was dependent on ulcer size with a minimum of 500 impulses at energy setting E2 (equivalent to 0.23 mJ/mm^2 energy flux density) at a rate of 4 shocks per second. Treatments were conducted two times per week totaling 6 treatments over 3 weeks duration. Study quality was rated as poor due to an inadequate method of allocation concealment and lack of blinding (patients and healthcare providers). Nine patients were excluded from the final analyses, two in the EST group due to poor compliance (not defined) and seven in the HBOT group due to incomplete follow-up data. The definition of a completely healed ulcer was not reported.

Completely healed ulcers were reported in 25% in the HBOT group versus 55% in the EST group (RR=0.46, 95% CI 0.25 to 0.84) after one course of therapy, four weeks for HBOT and three weeks for EST. No ulcers worsened in either group but there were significantly more unchanged ulcers in the HBOT group compared to the EST group, 60% versus 11%, respectively. Twenty-seven patients (EST 12 patients/14 feet and HBOT 15/17 feet) with improved but incomplete healing received a second course of treatment four-to-six weeks from the first treatment. Only one ulcer of 17 (6%) completely healed in the HBOT group compared to seven of 14 (50%) ulcers in the EST group (p=0.005). Four patients receiving HBOT developed middle ear barotraumas and sinus pain. No adverse events were reported in the EST group.

Ozone-Oxygen Therapy

One fair quality, double-blinded trial compared ozone-oxygen therapy to sham (placebo) for diabetic foot ulcers of at least 8 weeks in duration at study initiation.[50] A total of 61 patients, 32 in the ozone group and 29 in the sham group, were randomized. Mean age was 63 years and the proportion of men was 62%. Patients with infected ulcers (but no gangrene or active osteomyelitis) were included with antibiotic treatment as needed. Those with an ABI less than 0.65 were excluded. Most patients had diabetes type 2 (97%) and the baseline ulcer size was slightly larger in the ozone group (4.9 cm^2) compared to the sham group (3.5 cm^2). The ulcers were Wagner classification stage 2/3 or stage 4 following debridement. Study duration was 24 weeks. Patients received treatment or sham for 12 weeks followed by another 12 weeks until wound assessment. In the ozone group, therapy was divided into two phases. The patients initially received treatment sessions with the Ozoter device (OZ Recovery Tecnologies, Ramat Gan, Israel) four times weekly up to 4 weeks, or until granulation appeared in 50% of the wound area. Gas concentrations were 96% oxygen and 4% ozone with intervals between treatments not to exceed 1 day in 5 days a week. In the second phase, the sessions were reduced to two times weekly to complete the 12 weeks of treatment, and gas concentration was altered to 98% oxygen and 2% ozone. The control group received sham treatments with the ozone device circulating air only. Each treatment session lasted 26 minutes. The method of allocation concealment was unclear. Patients and investigators were blinded to mode of therapy. The intention-to-treat analyses included all enrolled patients and study withdrawals were adequately described. A per-protocol analysis, including only "completers," was also conducted.

After 24 weeks there was no statistically significant difference in the proportion of patients with completely healed wounds between the ozone group and sham group. In the ozone group, 41% of the patients had full wound closure versus 33% in the sham group (p=0.34). A large percentage of the study population discontinued prematurely, 16 (50%) in the ozone group and 11 (38%) in the sham group (p=0.44). When the analysis was limited to completers (n=34, 56% of the patients), complete wound closure was reported in 81% of the ozone group compared to 44% of the sham group (p=0.03). Post-hoc subgroup findings in patients with ulcers of 5 cm^2 or less found that active treatment resulted in 100% closure compared to 50% in the sham treatment group (p=0.006).

No differences were reported between active and sham therapy for ulcers infected during treatment, amputation, or withdrawals due to adverse events. Seven patients withdrew from the trial due to adverse events or complications, five in the ozone group and two in the sham group. Adverse events or complications in the ozone group included osteomyelitis, fever, wound infection, and pulmonary congestion. Events in the sham group included amputation and infection.

Summary of Key Question 1

Nine different advanced wound care therapies used for treatment of diabetic ulcers provided information on our primary and secondary outcomes. Most compared outcomes to standard care, placebo or sham treatments with few reporting comparative effectiveness findings versus other advanced wound care therapies. Advanced wound care therapies included collagen, biological dressings, biological skin equivalents, platelet-derived growth factors, platelet-rich plasma, silver products, negative pressure wound therapy, hyperbaric oxygen therapy, and ozone-oxygen therapy. We summarize our primary and secondary outcome findings below. We found insufficient evidence to address the question whether efficacy and comparative effectiveness differed according to patient demographics, comorbid conditions, treatment compliance, or activity level.

Primary Outcomes

Advanced wound care therapies using platelet-rich plasma or ozone oxygen therapy did not improve diabetic ulcer healing compared to standard care (2 studies) or another advanced care therapy (1 study). Other therapies provided mixed results. Four studies compared collagen products to standard care with only one study reporting significantly better healing in the collagen group (70% versus 46%, p=0.03). Pooled results from three studies indicate that the biological skin equivalent Dermagraft compared to standard care results in a non-significant improvement in ulcer healing favoring Dermagraft (35% versus 24%, low strength of evidence, see Executive Summary Table 1). We found moderate strength of evidence that the biological skin equivalent, bi-layer Apligraf, improved healing compared to standard care (55% versus 34%; p=0.001; 2 studies). While pooled results from studies of platelet-derived growth factor showed improvement in the percentage of ulcers healed compared to placebo or standard care (58% versus 37%; p=0.04; 7 studies) the strength of evidence was low due to high heterogeneity of results between studies. One good quality study provided moderate strength evidence that negative pressure wound therapy improved healing more than standard care (43% versus 29%, p<0.05). Three long-term, fair quality studies of HBOT reported significantly better healing with HBOT (52% to 66%) than sham therapy or standard care (0% to 29%).

Few studies reported time to ulcer healing and other primary outcomes. We found no benefit in time to ulcer healing for collagen, biological dressings, or silver products. We found mixed but generally negative results for biological skin equivalents (1 of 4 Dermagraft and 1 of 3 Apligraf studies showing benefit compared to standard care), platelet-derived growth factors (4 of 8 studies reporting showing benefit compared to placebo or standard care), platelet-rich plasma (1 of 2 studies showing benefit compared to another advanced therapy), and negative pressure wound therapy (1 of 3 studies showing benefit compared to standard care). Strength of evidence was low or insufficient for all findings related to time to ulcer healing. One study of a silver dressing versus a calcium dressing reported a global outcome of healed or improved ulcers with no difference between groups. No studies reported on return to daily activities.

Secondary Outcomes

The most commonly reported secondary outcomes were ulcers infected during treatment and ulcer recurrence. No study reported a benefit for these outcomes for any of the advanced therapies reviewed. Fewer amputations were reported in three studies (one each of a biological skin equivalent, negative pressure wound therapy, and hyperbaric oxygen therapy all compared to standard care) while five studies reported no difference. Few studies reported other secondary outcomes of interest including revascularization or surgery, pain or discomfort, hospitalization, need for home care, or quality of life. No significant differences between treatment groups (including 12 studies comparing an advanced therapy to standard care, 3 studies comparing one advanced therapy to another advanced therapy, and 1 study with both standard therapy and advanced therapy comparison arms) were seen in all-cause mortality though studies were not designed to assess this outcome. We found no significant differences in study withdrawals due to adverse events or allergic reactions to treatment.

.

Table 11. Strength of Evidence - Advanced Wound Care Therapies for Diabetic Ulcers

Treatment	Control(s)	Outcome	Number of Studies (n for Primary Outcome)*	Comments	Strength of Evidence
Collagen	Standard care	Percentage of ulcers healed	4 (483)	One study reported significant improvement compared to standard care. Three studies reported no significant difference between collagen and standard care. Trials were rated as fair quality.	Low
		Mean time to ulcer healing		One trial found a significant difference favoring standard care; two found no difference.	Low
Biological Dressings	Advanced therapy control (PDGF, BSE)	Percentage of ulcers healed	2 (99)	Two fair quality trials showed no difference compared to other advanced wound care therapies.	Low
		Mean time to ulcer healing		No trial was significantly different versus control.	Low
Biological Skin Equivalents [BSE] - Dermagraft	Standard care	Percentage of ulcers healed	3 (505)	A trend toward statistically significant improvement compared to standard care (RR=1.49, 95% CI 0.96 to 2.32, I²=43%). Trials were rated as fair quality.	Low
		Mean time to ulcer healing		Inconsistent results, with one trial reporting a significant difference versus standard care. Trials were rated as fair quality.	Low
BSE -Apligraf	Standard care	Percentage of ulcers healed	2 (279)	Two trials of fair quality found statistically significant improvement versus standard care (RR=1.58, 95% CI 1.20 to 2.08, I²=0%).	Moderate
		Mean time to ulcer healing		One trial reported a significant difference between Apligraf and standard care.	Low
BSE -Apligraf	Advanced therapy control (Skin allografts -Theraskin)	Percentage of ulcers healed	1 (29 ulcers)	One fair quality trial found no significant difference versus Theraskin.	Low
		Mean time to ulcer healing		No significant difference versus Theraskin.	Low
Platelet Derived Wound Healing [PDGF]	Placebo /standard care	Percentage of ulcers healed	7 (685)	Overall statistically significant improvement versus placebo (RR 1.45 [95% CI 1.03 to 2.05]) but results were inconsistent (I² 85%). Overall study quality was rated as fair.	Low
		Mean time to ulcer healing	5 (731)	Overall, PDGF demonstrated shorter duration of time to ulcer healing versus placebo.	Low
PDGF	Advanced therapy control (BSE, silver, sodium carboxy-methylcellulose)	Percentage of ulcers healed	3 (189)	No significant differences compared to an advanced therapy comparator. Trials were rated as fair quality.	Low
		Mean time to ulcer healing		No significant differences compared to an advanced therapy comparator.	Low
Platelet-Rich Plasma [PRP]	Placebo gel, Platelet-Poor Plasma	Percentage of ulcers healed	2 (96)	Neither of the studies (fair to poor quality) demonstrated a significant difference between PRP and its respective control.	Low
		Mean time to ulcer healing		Significantly shorter healing time compared to platelet-poor plasma. No significant difference versus placebo gel.	Low

Advanced Wound Care Therapies for Non-Healing Diabetic, Venous, and Arterial Ulcers: A Systematic Review

Treatment	Control(s)	Outcome	Number of Studies (n for Primary Outcome)*	Comments	Strength of Evidence
Silver Products	Standard care or advanced therapy controls (*calcium-based dressing, oak bark extract, polyherbal cream*)	Percentage of ulcers healed	4 (280)	One trial found silver ointment more effective than standard care. Two trials found no difference in healing between a silver cream or dressing and another advanced care product. Studies were of fair quality.	Low
		Mean time to ulcer healing	2 (174)	Two trials found no difference between silver and another advanced wound care product.	Low
Negative Pressure Wound Therapy [NPWT]	Standard care (*Advanced moist wound therapy, saline gauze*)	Percentage of ulcers healed	1 (335)	One trial of good quality found 43% in the NPWT group experienced ulcer healing compared to 29% treated with standard care (RR=1.49, 95% CI 1.11 to 2.01).	Moderate
		Mean time to ulcer healing	3 (432)	Results for time to healing were inconsistent based on 3 trials of mixed quality.	Low
Hyperbaric Oxygen Therapy (HBOT)	Sham or standard care	Percentage of ulcers healed	4 (233)	Three long-term studies of fair quality found significant improvement with adjunctive HBOT versus sham or standard care; one short-term study found no difference.	Low
		Mean time to ulcer healing	-	Outcome not reported.	Insufficient
HBOT	Advanced therapy control (*Extracorporeal shockwave therapy*)	Percentage of ulcers healed	1 (84)	One trial of poor quality found adjunctive HBOT less effective than extracorporeal shockwave therapy.	Low
		Mean time to ulcer healing	-	Outcome not reported.	Insufficient
Ozone-Oxygen Therapy	Sham	Percentage of ulcers healed	1 (61)	One trial of fair quality found no significant difference between ozone-oxygen and sham.	Low
		Mean time to ulcer healing	-	Outcome not reported.	Insufficient

*Number of ulcers evaluated for the primary outcome

The evidence is rated using the following grades: (1) high strength indicates further research is very unlikely to change the confidence in the estimate of effect, meaning that the evidence reflects the true effect; (2) moderate strength denotes further research may change our confidence in the estimate of effect and may change the estimate; (3) low strength indicates further research is very likely to have an important impact on the confidence in the estimate of effect and is likely to change the estimate, meaning there is low confidence that the evidence reflects the true effect; and (4) insufficient, indicating that the evidence is unavailable or does not permit a conclusion.

KEY QUESTION #2. What are the efficacy and harms of therapies for venous ulcers? Is efficacy dependent on ancillary therapies? Does efficacy differ according to patient demographics, comorbid conditions, treatment compliance, or activity level?

Overview of Studies

Table 12 contains an overview of studies of therapies for venous ulcers.[52-72] Twenty trials (in 22 articles) met eligibility criteria including 1 trial of collagen (n=73), 1 trial of biological dressings (n=120), 3 trials of biological skin equivalents (n=380), 4 trials of keratinocytes (n=502), 1 trial of platelet-rich plasma (n=86), 6 trials of silver products (n=771), 1 trial of intermittent pneumatic compression therapy (n=54), 2 trials of electromagnetic therapy (n=63), and 1 trial of hyperbaric oxygen therapy (n=16). Sixteen trials compared an advanced wound care therapy to standard care or placebo. In four trials, the comparator was a different advanced therapy.

Overall, the mean age of study participants ranged from 56 to 73 years and 26% to 61% were male. In 5 studies reporting race, 62% to 100% were white, 0% to 33% were black, 0% to 6% were Hispanic, and 0% to 2% were Asian. Mean ulcer sizes ranged from 1.2 to 11.1 cm^2 with ulcer durations of 7 to 626 weeks.

In 14 trials, the ulcer was described as a "leg" ulcer (with 1 trial specifying the location as medial distal one-third of the leg). In 2 trials, the ulcer was described as a "lower extremity" ulcer (with 1 trial specifying that 80% of the ulcers were on the angle or calf). Three trials did not report the ulcer location describing the ulcer only as a "venous ulcer." In 12 trials, the diagnosis of venous ulcer was based on clinical signs or symptoms of venous insufficiency. The remaining 8 trials required either patients to have adequate arterial circulation or specifically excluded patients with known arterial insufficiency.

Collagen

One fair quality RCT enrolled 73 patients with a venous leg ulcer and followed them over twelve weeks of treatment with Promogran or standard wound care.[52] Standard care included compression therapy. Participants in the study had an average age of 73 years; 35 percent were males. Patients with infected ulcers and ulcers linked to diabetes were excluded; an ABI of greater than 0.8 was required for inclusion. The trial did not include a run-in period with standard care and compliance with treatment was not reported. The mean ulcer size was 8.2 cm^2 and the mean ulcer duration was 9.2 months. The study reported no significant difference between treatment arms in ulcer size, ulcer duration, or ancillary therapies. Demographic and ulcer characteristics are reported in Appendix D, Table 1.

Primary Outcomes (Appendix D, Table 2)

The percentage of venous ulcers healed by study completion did not differ significantly between the Promogran and standard wound care groups (49% versus 33%, p=0.18; ARD=16%, 95% CI -7% to 38%).[52] The effects of patient factors or ancillary therapies on outcomes were not reported.

Secondary Outcomes (Appendix D, Tables 3, 4, and 5)

Significantly fewer ulcers were infected during treatment with collagen compared to standard care (0% versus 14%, p=0.03). No significant differences between collagen and standard care were noted for the percentage of withdrawals due to adverse events or percentage of patients having an allergic reaction to treatment.[52]

Biological Dressings

One study, enrolling 120 patients,[53] compared OASIS Wound Matrix plus compression therapy to compression therapy alone (standard care) in treatment of chronic leg ulcers unresponsive to standard therapy. This industry-sponsored study was of fair quality and took place in multiple sites across the United States, United Kingdom, and Canada. Patients with infected ulcers, uncontrolled diabetes, or an ABI less than 0.8 were excluded. Compliance with treatment was not reported. The average ulcer size at baseline was 11.1 cm². The mean age of the patients was 64 years, 42% were male, and 81% were white. Thirty-four percent of ulcers were present for 1 to 3 months; 37% were present for more than 12 months. Additional study characteristics are presented in Appendix D, Table 1.

Primary Outcomes (Appendix D, Table 2)

Treatment with OASIS resulted in a statistically significant improvement in incidence of ulcer healing, with 55% of treated patients achieving complete healing at 12 weeks, versus 34% in the standard care group (ARD=20%, 95% CI 3% to 38%; p=0.02) but not at 6 months (67% versus 46%, p=ns).[53]

Debridement was only performed if deemed clinically necessary. This allowed for covariate and subgroup analysis comparing those who received baseline debridement to those who did not. Covariate analysis showed that OASIS had a consistently higher rate of healing compared to standard care regardless of debridement status, but subgroup analysis found the difference between study groups was exaggerated in patients who received baseline debridement. Sixty-three percent of OASIS patients who underwent baseline debridement healed at 12 weeks, versus 30% of standard care patients who received initial debridement (p=0.02).[53] Covariate analysis also showed the higher incidence of healing with OASIS was consistently observed when accounting for the presence of vascular disease (p=0.03), type 2 diabetes (p=0.02), endocrine disease (p=0.03), and hypertension (p=0.02).

Secondary Outcomes (Appendix D, Tables 3, 4, and 5)

At 6 months follow-up, there was a significant difference in recurrence (0% of healed ulcers originally treated with OASIS versus 30% of healed ulcers in the standard care arm, p=0.03). There was no difference between groups in ulcers infected during treatment. Two patients in the OASIS group were hospitalized and unable to complete the study versus none in the standard care group (p=ns).[53] No statistically significant differences between treatment groups were reported for withdrawals due to adverse events, proportion of patients with adverse events, all-cause mortality, or allergic reaction to treatment.

Table 12. Overview of Therapies for Venous Ulcers

Study, year	N Randomized	Treatment	Product	Comparator	Healed ulcers	Mean time to ulcer healing	Global assessment	Return to daily activities	Ulcers infected during treatment	Amputation	Revascularization/surgery	Recurrence	Time to recurrence	Pain/discomfort	Hospitalization	Required home care	Quality of life	Withdrawals due to adverse events	Patients with ≥ 1 adverse event	All-cause mortality	Allergic reactions to treatment
Vin 2002[52]	73	Col	Promogran	Non-adherent	-				+					-				-			-
Mostow 2005[53]	120	BD	OASIS	Compression bandage	+				-			+			-			-	-	-	±
Falanga 1998[54]	309	BSE	Apligraf	Compression bandage	+	+			-			-		-				-		-	
Falanga 1999[55] (subset of Falanga 1998; pts with ulcer duration > 1 yr)	120	BSE	Apligraf	Compression bandage	+	+						-									
Krishnamoorthy 2003[56]	53	BSE	Dermagraft	Compression bandage	-				-									-	±	-	
Omar 2004[57]	18	BSE	Dermagraft	Compression bandage	-																
Lindgren 1998[58]	27	Keratinocyte	Keratinocyte sheets + pneumatic compression therapy	Pneumatic compression therapy	-																
Navratilova 2004[59]	50	Keratinocyte	Cryopreserved keratinocytes	Lyophilized keratinocytes	-	-															
Harding 2005[60]	200	Keratinocyte	Keratinocytes	Vehicle + std care or std care only	-	-			-			-		-	-						-
Vanscheidt 2007[61]	225	Keratinocyte	Keratinocytes (autologous)	Compression bandage	+	+														-	
Stacey 2000[62]	86	PRP	Platelet lysate	Placebo	-														-	-	
Belcaro 2010[38]	82	Silver Ointment	Aidance	Standard	+									-					-	-	-
Bishop 1992[63]	93	Tri-peptide Copper Complex		Silver Cream (Silvadene) or Tri-peptide placebo	→*		+					-		-					-	-	

58

Advanced Wound Care Therapies for Non-Healing Diabetic, Venous, and Arterial Ulcers: A Systematic Review

Study, year	N Randomized	Treatment	Product	Comparator	Healed ulcers	Mean time to ulcer healing	Global assessment	Return to daily activities	Ulcers infected during treatment	Amputation	Revascularization/ surgery	Recurrence	Time to recurrence	Pain/discomfort	Hospitalization	Required home care	Quality of life	Withdrawals due to adverse events	Patients with ≥ 1 adverse event	All-cause mortality	Allergic reactions to treatment
Blair 1988[64]	60	Silver Cream	Flamazine	Non-adherent + Non-occlusive dressing	-																-
Dimakakos 2009[65]	42	Silver Dressing		Standard	+	±								±							
Harding 2011[66]	281	Ionic Silver Dressing	AQUA-CEL	Lipidocolloid silver	-		+														
Michaels 2009a, b[67,68]	213	Silver Dressing	6 options	Non-silver dressing	-	-			-			-					-	-	-	-	
Schuler 1996[69]	54	IPC		Unna's Boot (Compression)	-									-				-			-
Ieran 1990[70]	44	EMT	Dermagan	Sham	+	±	-	-	±			-		-				-		-	
Kenkre 1996[71]	19	EMT	Elmedistraal	Sham	-			±	-					+				-		-	-
Hammarlund 1994[72]	16	HBOT		Sham	-													-			

BD – Biological Dressing; BSE – Biological Skin Equivalent; Col – Collagen; EMT – Electromagnetic therapy; EST – Extracorporeal Shock Wave Therapy; HBOT – Hyperbaric Oxygen Therapy; IPC – Intermittent Pneumatic Compression Therapy; NaCMC - Sodium Carboxymethylcellulose; NPWT – Negative Pressure Wound Therapy; PDGF – Platelet-derived Growth Factor; PRP – Platelet Rich Plasma

+ Treatment group better than comparator (p< 0.05)
- Treatment group demonstrated no significant benefit
→ Treatment group worse than comparator
± Significance could not be determined
* (+ for silver)

Biological Skin Equivalents

We identified three RCTs related to the use of biological skin equivalents in ulcers of venous etiology. Two studies evaluated the use of Dermagraft for ulcers described only as "leg" ulcers. One study evaluated the use of Apligraf but did not describe the ulcer location. The comparator in all three studies was standard care including compression bandages. One Dermagraft study was a small (n=18), single center trial of fair quality that was done in the UK.[57] No study sponsor was reported. The other Dermagraft study was a small (n=53), industry sponsored trial of fair quality that took place in six centers across the UK and Canada.[56] Both studies allowed ulcers with an initial area of 3 to 25 cm² and took place over a period of 12 weeks. The Apligraf study was a large (n=309), industry-sponsored study of fair quality, which took place at 15 sites across the U.S.[54] The average ulcer size in this study was significantly smaller than the other studies, with a mean ulcer area of 1.2 cm² at baseline. This trial followed patients for 6 months. None of the studies reported compliance with standard care. None reported differences between study arms at baseline but one did not report a statistical analysis.[56] No study enrolled patients with infected ulcers; only one reported allowing antibiotics as needed.[56] All of the studies excluded patients with arterial insufficiency. One included a 14 day run-in period with compression.[56] Summary baseline data are presented in Table 13. Additional information about the studies is presented in Appendix D, Table 1.

Table 13. Baseline Study Characteristics: Biological Skin Equivalents

Characteristic	Number of Studies Reporting	Mean (unless noted)	Range
Number of Patients Randomized	3	380 total	18 - 309
Age	3	62	60 - 69
Gender (% male)	3	51	42 - 61
Race/Ethnicity (%)			
White	2	79	76 - 94
Black	2	16	4 - 18
Other	2	5	2 - 5
BMI	1	30.4	30.4
ABI	2[a]	1.1	1.06 - 1.1
Ulcer Size (cm²)	3	2.5	1.2 - 10.7
Ulcer Duration	3[b]		
Study Duration (weeks)	3	9	8 - 12

[a]Mean/median ABI not reported in one study, but all participants were >0.65 by exclusion criteria
[b]All 3 studies reported ulcer duration in a different format: Krishnamoorthy 2003:[56] *median* duration of 47.7 *days*; Omar, 2004:[57] *mean* duration of 119.3 *weeks*; Falanga, 1998:[54] <6 months: 30.6%, 6-12 months: 21.1%, 1-2 years: 13.8%, >2 years: 34.5%

Primary Outcomes (Appendix D, Table 2)

In two small studies of Dermagraft, there was no significant difference in healed ulcers compared to standard care.[56,57] Pooled results are presented in Figure 8. The overall risk ratio was 2.96 (95% CI 0.93 to 9.44, I²=0%). The large trial using Apligraf did show a significant benefit compared to standard compression bandage therapy for incidence of complete ulcer healing at 6 months (63% versus 49%; ARD=14%, 95% CI 3% to 26%; p=0.02) and median time to closure (61 days versus 181 days, p=0.003).[54] A similar pattern was observed when only ulcers of greater than 1 year duration were considered.[55] Additional subgroup analyses from this trial found significant differences in treatment efficacy for certain patient subpopulations. In ulcers with a duration less than 6 months at the beginning of the study time to ulcer healing did not differ significantly between biological skin equivalent and standard care. In ulcers present for over 6 months, significantly more rapid healing was observed in the biological skin equivalent group (median of 92 days versus 190 days for control, p=0.001). Similarly, a significant benefit in time to closure was seen for biological skin equivalent compared to standard compression bandage therapy in patients with deeper ulcers (83 days versus 183 days, p=0.003). Stratification by initial ulcer area found that Apligraf significantly improved ulcer healing (p<0.05) when used in both large (defined as greater than 1000 mm^2) and small ulcers.[54] The effect of ancillary therapies on treatment efficacy could not be assessed from any of the studies.

Figure 8. Proportion of Venous Ulcers Healed - Biological Skin Equivalent (Dermagraft) versus Compression Bandage

Study or Subgroup	Dermagraft Events	Total	Control Events	Total	Weight	Risk Ratio M-H, Random, 95% CI	Risk Ratio M-H, Random, 95% CI
Krishnamoorthy 2003	5	13	2	13	64.1%	2.50 [0.59, 10.64]	
Omar 2004	5	10	1	8	35.9%	4.00 [0.58, 27.70]	
Total (95% CI)		23		21	100.0%	2.96 [0.93, 9.44]	
Total events	10		3				

Heterogeneity: Tau² = 0.00; Chi² = 0.15, df = 1 (P = 0.70); I² = 0%
Test for overall effect: Z = 1.83 (P = 0.07)

0.05 0.2 1 5 20
Favors Control Favors Dermagraft

*Kishnamoorthy 2003 – Analysis is for Group 2 (4 pieces of Dermagraft applied on day 0, and weeks 1, 4, and 8) versus compression bandage

Secondary Outcomes (Appendix D, Tables 3, 4, and 5)

Two studies, one of Dermagraft[56] and one of Apligraf[54] reported no difference between treatment with biological skin equivalent or standard compression bandage therapy in the incidence of infection. The Apligraf study also reported no difference in the incidence of cellulitis.[54] Rate of recurrence was reported in the Apligraf study. No significant difference was seen in the percentage of ulcers recurring within one year (12% versus 16% of control patients)[54] with similar findings for the subgroup with ulcers of greater than 1 year duration.[55] In the Apligraf study, there was also no difference in pain between treatment groups.[54] Of the two studies that reported adverse events, both reported no differences between biological skin equivalent and standard compression bandage therapy in withdrawals due to adverse events.[54,56] There was also no difference in all-cause mortality. One study reported no difference in the incidence of adverse events or serious adverse events.[56] No instances of immune intolerance or reactivity to grafts were reported.

Keratinocytes

Four RCTs met eligibility criteria and looked at the use of keratinocytes in venous ulcers. Three studies described the ulcers only as "leg" ulcers; one specified the location as medial distal one-third of the leg.[58] These trials had marked heterogeneity across several important parameters: keratinocyte source (autologous or allogeneic); cellular state of keratinocytes (fresh, frozen, or lysed); comparators (other keratinocyte product, standard of care); and study size, protocols, and quality. This variability hampered aggregation and the ability to generalize results. The four studies consisted of the following: a large, multinational study of fair quality that took place in Belgium, Germany, Poland, and the UK[60] (n=200); a large, multinational study of fair quality that took place in Hungary, Germany, and the Czech Republic[61] (n=225); a smaller study of poor quality that took place at a single site in the Czech Republic[59] (n=50); and a small study of fair quality that took place in Sweden[58] (n=27). Inclusion criteria for ulcer size varied. One study included ulcers between 1 and 20 cm²; the median size was 5.2 cm².[60] Another study included ulcers of 2 to 50 cm² with 60% of the study ulcers between 2 and 10 cm² and 39% over 10 cm².[61] The third study included ulcers greater than 2 cm² and the mean ulcer size was 10.7 cm².[59] In the last study, all ulcers were greater than 2 cm² with a mean ulcer size of 8.4 cm².[58] One study reported having industry sponsorship;[60] the other studies did not include financial disclosures. One study reported study compliance and identified protocol violations in 5.3%.[60] Three of the studies either excluded patients with infection or required treatment before study entry; one did not report infection status.[61] Two studies reported antibiotic use during the study, either for cellulitis[58] or prior to graft placement, if infection was present.[59] All of the studies excluded patients with arterial insufficiency; one study excluded patients with diabetic ulcers.[60] None of the studies reported significant differences between study arms at baseline. Two of the studies included a run-in period with standard care, either 2 weeks[61] or 4 weeks.[60] Summary baseline characteristics are reported in Table 14. Additional study characteristics are presented in Appendix D, Table 1.

Table 14. Baseline Study Characteristics: Keratinocytes

Characteristic	Number of Studies Reporting	Mean (unless noted)	Range
Number of Patients Randomized	4	502 total	27 - 225
Age	2[a]	66	63 - 67
Gender (% male)	4	38	33 - 39
Race/Ethnicity (%)	1		
White	1	100	-
BMI	2[b]	28.9	28.6 - 30.1
Smoking (%)	1	19.1	-
ABI	2[c]		
Ulcer Size (cm²)	2[d]	9.2	6.3 - 10.7
Ulcer Duration (weeks)	1[e]	102.7	-
Study Duration (weeks)	4	23	8 - 26
History of DM	1	6%	-

[a]Two additional studies reported median ages of 76 years and 67.5 years
[b]One additional study reported median BMI of 28.9
[c]Two studies reported median ABI of 1.0 and 1.1; all patients in 2 other studies had ABI >0.8 per exclusion criteria
[d]Two other studies reported ulcer size using other formats: Harding, 2005:[60] median ulcer size=5.2 cm²; Vanscheidt, 2007:[61] ulcer size 2-10 cm²: 60.4%; ulcer size >10 cm²: 38.7%
[e]3 additional studies reported ulcer duration in other formats: Harding, 2005:[60] *median* duration of 43 weeks; Lindgren, 1998:[58] <2 years: 44.4%, >2 years: 55.6%; Vanscheidt, 2007:[61] 3-12 months: 59.1%, >12 months: 40.9%

Primary Outcomes (Appendix D, Table 2)

One trial demonstrated significant improvements in both proportion of ulcers healed (38% versus 22%, p=0.01) and median time to complete healing (176 days versus more than 201 days, p<0.0001) when BioSeed-S (autologous keratinocytes in fibrin sealant) was compared to standard compression bandage therapy. In subgroups of patients with ulcers of 12 months or less, greater than 12 months, 2 to 10 cm^2, or greater than 10 cm^2, the proportion of ulcers healed was significantly greater in the keratinocyte group only for patients with larger ulcers at baseline (greater than 10 cm^2). Time to ulcer healing was significantly higher for patients treated with keratinocytes in all of the subgroups.[61] In other studies, no statistical differences in ulcer healing were seen when cryopreserved, cultured epidermal allografts (CEA) were compared with pneumatic compression therapy,[58] when cryopreserved CEA were compared to lyophilized CEA,[59] and when lyophilized keratinocytes were compared to a combined control group of standard compression therapy and standard therapy plus keratinocyte vehicle.[60] Pooled ulcer healing results for the two studies comparing keratinocyte treatment to standard care (with compression therapy) are presented in Figure 9. The absolute risk difference was 14%, 95% CI 5% to 23%. The overall risk ratio was 1.57 (95% CI 1.16 to 2.11, I^2=0%) indicating a significant overall benefit of keratinocyte therapy compared to standard care. Two studies reported time to healing with no differences between treatment groups in either study, one a comparison of keratinocytes to standard care,[60] the other a comparison to another advanced therapy.[59] No comparisons could be made within or between studies regarding the effect of ancillary therapies on treatment efficacy.

Figure 9. Proportion of Venous Ulcers Healed - Keratinocytes versus Standard Care

Study or Subgroup	Keratinocytes Events	Total	Standard Care Events	Total	Weight	Risk Ratio M-H, Random, 95% CI	Risk Ratio M-H, Random, 95% CI
Harding 2005	36	95	26	98	50.6%	1.43 [0.94, 2.17]	
Vanscheidt 2007	44	116	24	109	49.4%	1.72 [1.13, 2.63]	
Total (95% CI)		211		207	100.0%	1.57 [1.16, 2.11]	
Total events	80		50				

Heterogeneity: Tau^2 = 0.00; Chi^2 = 0.38, df = 1 (P = 0.54); I^2 = 0%
Test for overall effect: Z = 2.96 (P = 0.003)

0.2 0.5 1 2 5
Favors Std. Care   Favors Keratinocytes

*Harding 2005 – Analysis is for the "as treated" ITT cohort.

Secondary Outcomes (Appendix D, Tables 3, 4, and 5)

Few secondary outcomes were reported. In one study, the percentage of ulcers infected during treatment, ulcer recurrence, and pain during treatment or follow-up did not differ between keratinocyte therapy and a combined (standard care and vehicle) control group.[60] Another study reported that pain was significantly reduced during the first week after treatment application with no difference between the two keratinocyte products.[59] Only the two large studies reported adverse events.[60,61] One study reported 65 events in 38 patients in the keratinocyte group and 51 events in 27 patients in the compression therapy group. Of the 116 patients receiving keratinocyte therapy, 1 experienced a minor adverse event "certainly" related to the treatment, 2 were "probably" related, and 6 were "possibly" related.[61] The other study reported no difference between advanced treatment and a combined standard care and vehicle control group in "burning, stinging, pain, or itching" sensations.[60] There was no difference in all-cause mortality between treatment groups in either study.

Platelet Rich Plasma (PRP)

One RCT enrolling 86 patients with ulcers described only as "leg" ulcers, compared the efficacy of PRP to placebo over 39 weeks.[62] This fair quality trial was conducted in Australia and funded by a combination of industry and government sources. Both groups received standard compression therapy. The authors did not report inclusion or exclusion criteria related to infection, whether there was a run-in period with standard care, or whether compliance with treatment was monitored. Patients were required to have an ABI greater than 0.9 for inclusion. The mean age of participants was 71 years; 42 percent were male. Mean ulcer size was 4.9 cm^2 and the mean ulcer duration prior to enrollment was 3 months. The study reported no significant difference between treatment arms in ulcer size, ulcer duration, or ancillary therapies. Treatments were applied twice weekly until wound healing or up to the 9 month study duration. Demographic and ulcer characteristics are reported in Appendix D, Table 1.

Primary Outcomes (Appendix D, Table 2)

There was no significant difference between PRP and placebo in the percentage of ulcers healed at study completion (79% versus 77%, p=ns).[62] Time to complete healing was not reported.

Secondary Outcomes (Appendix D, Tables 3, 4, and 5)

Two hospitalizations leading to study withdrawal were reported but the treatment group the patients were assigned to was not provided. There were 6 withdrawals from the study due to adverse events (5 with allergy to the paste bandage and 1 with leg trauma related to the bandages) but the treatment group was not reported.[62]

Silver Products

We identified six studies of silver products used to treat venous ulcers.[38,63-68] Two studies compared a silver dressing to a dressing without silver,[65,67,68] two compared silver ointment to standard care,[38,60] one compared silver cream to a tri-peptide copper cream or tri-peptide placebo (with silver as the control treatment),[63] and one compared an ionic silver dressing to a lipidocolloid silver dressing.[66] The studies were conducted in the United States,[63] the United Kingdom,[64,67,68] Greece,[65] Italy,[38] and Europe.[66] Enrollments ranged from 42 to 281 with a total enrollment of 771. Two studies were of good quality[64,66] and four were of fair quality. A summary of study characteristics is presented in Table 15 with additional information about the studies in Appendix D, Table 1.

Table 15. Summary of Baseline Characteristics: Silver Products

Characteristic	Number of Studies Reporting	Mean (unless noted)	Range
Number of Patients Randomized	6	771 total	42 - 281
Age (years)	6	65.6	47 - 71
Gender (% male)	5	41.6	35 - 50
Race/Ethnicity (%)			
White	1	62	-
Black	1	33	-
Other	1	5	-
BMI	1	30	-
Smoking, Current (%)	2	22.7	18.3 - 33.7
ABI	1	1.04	-
Ulcer Size (cm²)	3[a]	6.0	3.2 - 10.5
Ulcer Duration (months)	3[b]	19.4	9.0 - 46.4
Infection (%)	4[c,d]	-	-
Study Duration (weeks)	6	8.6	4 - 12
History of Diabetes (%)	2[e]	9	-
History of MI or Cardiac Failure (%)	1	14	-
History of Stroke or TIA (%)	1	8	-

[a]One study reported that 72% were <3 cm diameter; another reported that 52% were <3 cm diameter
[b]One study reported that 38.5% were >12 weeks
[c]Three studies reported excluding 1) >10⁵ bacteria/gram of tissue, systemic sepsis or bone infection; 2) clinically infected ulcers or receiving local or systemic antibiotics (included ulcers with at least 3 of the following: pain, perilesional skin erythema, edema, foul odor, or high levels of exudate); or 3) receiving oral or parenteral antibiotics
[d]One study included only patients with infected ulcers
[e]One study excluded patients with diabetes

Ulcers were described as "leg" ulcers in 3 studies[64,65,67,68] and lower extremity ulcers in 1 study.[63] One study did not specify ulcer location[38] and one reported that 47% were ankle, 33% calf, 18% gaiter, and 2% foot ulcers.[66] Three studies excluded patients with signs of infection or patients who were receiving antibiotics;[63,66-68] all patients had infected ulcers in two studies,[64,64] and one did not report infection status.[38] Only one reported use of antibiotics, as needed.[65] All trials excluded patients with arterial insufficiency. None of the trials included a run-in period with standard care. Compression bandaging was part of standard care in all of the trials; one trial reported monitoring compliance with treatment but did not provide results based on compliance.[63] Four studies reported no baseline differences between treatment groups while one noted gender distribution and height varied (not found to be related to outcomes),[63] and one found differences in BMI and ulcer location (right versus left leg).[67,68] Two studies reported mean ulcer sizes of 3.2 cm²[(38)]and 3.4 cm².[64] The latter study included only ulcers up to 10 cm². One study reported a mean ulcer size of 10.5 cm² with ulcers of 3 cm² to 50 cm² included in the trial.[63] Another study included ulcers between 5 cm² to 40 cm² but did not report a mean size.[60] One study reported that 72% of the study ulcers were less than 3 cm in diameter[67,68] and a second study reported that 52% were less than 3 cm in diameter.[65] Ulcer duration was reported in 4 studies. In three studies, the mean ulcer duration ranged from 9 months to 46.4 months.[64-66] In the fourth study, only ulcers of greater than 6 weeks were included; 38.5% were of greater than 12 weeks.[67,68] The studies were designed to address effectiveness and safety with one looking at non-inferiority of a new silver product.[66]

Primary Outcomes (Appendix D, Table 2)

All six studies reported ulcer healing. Two studies found significantly greater rates of healing in the silver cream/ointment groups at 4 weeks when compared to standard care (42% versus 22%, p<0.05)[38] or to copper cream (21% versus 0%, p=0.01).[63] No difference was found between silver cream and the copper cream placebo (31% versus 3%, p=0.05).[63] One study comparing silver cream to a non-adherent and non-occlusive dressing found no benefit for the silver cream at 12 weeks (63% versus 80%).[64] Pooled results from three studies (Figure 10) showed no statistically significant difference in ulcer healing with silver cream (range 21% to 63%) versus standard care or placebo copper cream (range 3% to 80%) with evidence of large heterogeneity (RR=1.65, 95% CI 0.54 to 5.03, I^2=84%).

One study found a higher rate of ulcer healing in the silver dressing group compared to standard care (non-silver dressing) at 9 weeks (81% versus 48%, p=0.02).[65] The two remaining studies found no difference at 8 weeks between two silver-based dressings (17% versus 15%)[66] and no differences at 12 weeks (60% versus 57%) or 1 year (96% in both groups) between a silver and a non-silver dressing.[67,68] Pooled data from two studies of silver versus non-silver dressings (Figure 10) again show no statistically significant difference with evidence of heterogeneity (RR=1.27, 95% CI 0.80 to 2.01, I^2=67%).

Two studies presented data on factors related to healing. In one study comparing silver to non-silver dressings, female gender (p=0.01) and smaller ulcer size (up to 3 cm versus above 3 cm; p=0.008) were significant predictors of healing at 12 weeks.[67,68] In the other study, the significant overall benefit of the silver dressing compared to standard care was also observed among the 30 study ulcers of less than 0.5 cm depth with 93% healing in the silver group versus 56% in the non-silver group (p=0.04). For ulcers greater than 0.5 cm depth (12 of the 42 study ulcers) there was no benefit of the silver dressing (57% versus 20%).[65] In the silver dressing group, 100% (6/6) of ulcers with a high degree of exudation were healed following treatment; in the non-silver group, none of 8 ulcers with a high degree of exudation were healed.[65]

Two studies, both comparing silver dressings to non-silver dressings, reported time to healing. One study found no difference between groups (medians of 67 [silver] and 58 [non-silver] days),[67,68] the other study reported mean times to healing of 6.1 weeks (silver) and 6.4 weeks (non-silver) but whether the difference was significant was not reported.[65] Silver cream was superior to tri-peptide copper cream in a composite measure of the degree of erythemia, exudation, and granulation[63] and an ionic silver dressing was superior to a lipidocolloid silver dressing in a composite outcome of healed or markedly improved ulcers.[66]

Figure 10. Proportion of Venous Ulcers Healed – Silver Products

Study or Subgroup	Silver Events	Total	Control Events	Total	Weight	Risk Ratio M-H, Random, 95% CI
3.1.1 Cream						
Belcaro 2010	19	44	8	38	38.4%	2.05 [1.02, 4.14]
Bishop 1992	6	28	1	29	17.9%	6.21 [0.80, 48.38]
Blair 1998	19	30	24	30	43.7%	0.79 [0.57, 1.10]
Subtotal (95% CI)		102		97	100.0%	1.65 [0.54, 5.03]
Total events	44		33			

Heterogeneity: Tau² = 0.71; Chi² = 12.22, df = 2 (P = 0.002); I² = 84%
Test for overall effect: Z = 0.88 (P = 0.38)

	Silver Events	Total	Control Events	Total	Weight	Risk Ratio M-H, Random, 95% CI
3.1.2 Silver cream versus copper cream						
Bishop 1992	6	28	0	29	100.0%	13.45 [0.79, 228.07]
Subtotal (95% CI)		28		29	100.0%	13.45 [0.79, 228.07]
Total events	6		0			

Heterogeneity: Not applicable
Test for overall effect: Z = 1.80 (P = 0.07)

	Silver Events	Total	Control Events	Total	Weight	Risk Ratio M-H, Random, 95% CI
3.1.3 Dressing						
Dimakakos 2009	17	21	10	21	39.3%	1.70 [1.04, 2.79]
Michaels 2009	62	104	59	104	60.7%	1.05 [0.83, 1.32]
Subtotal (95% CI)		125		125	100.0%	1.27 [0.80, 2.01]
Total events	79		69			

Heterogeneity: Tau² = 0.08; Chi² = 2.99, df = 1 (P = 0.08); I² = 67%
Test for overall effect: Z = 1.01 (P = 0.31)

Favors Control   Favors Silver

Test for subgroup differences: Chi² = 2.71, df = 2 (P = 0.26), I² = 26.2%

Secondary Outcomes (Appendix D, Tables 3, 4, and 5)

One study reported on ulcers infected during treatment with no difference between an ionic silver dressing (11%) and a lipidocolloid silver dressing (9%).[66] Two studies reported on ulcer recurrence. In one study, no difference was observed in recurrence between ulcers treated with a silver dressing versus a non-silver dressing (12% versus 14%).[67,68] Another study reported that 17% of the ulcers treated with silver cream recurred. There were no healed ulcers in the tri-peptide copper cream group and the one healed ulcer in the tri-peptide placebo cream group did not recur.[63] Pain was assessed in three studies, one comparing silver cream to tri-peptide copper cream,[63] one comparing an ionic silver dressing to a lipidocolloid silver dressing,[66] and one comparing a silver dressing to a non-silver dressing.[65] No differences between treatment groups were observed in the two studies comparing advanced wound therapies.[63,66] In the third study, it was reported that 100% of patients in the silver dressing group were pain-free by the end of the eighth week of treatment; 62% of the standard care (non-silver dressing) patients were pain-free after 9 weeks of treatment.[65] Quality of life was reported in one study, a comparison of silver and non-silver dressings. No difference was found between groups at either 12 weeks (post-treatment) or 1 year.[67,68] Study withdrawals due to adverse events were documented in three studies with no differences between silver cream and standard care,[38] two silver dressings,[66] or silver and non-silver dressings.[67,68] In one study, there were no withdrawals and no adverse events.[38] In the second study, the percentages of patients withdrawing were 6% (ionic silver dressing group) and 9% (lipidocolloid silver dressing group).[66] Overall adverse event rates were 50% and 42%, respectively; study-related adverse event rates were 23% and 18%. The third study reported one withdrawal in the silver dressing group.[67,68] No differences were observed between two silver dressings or a silver and a non-silver dressing in all-cause mortality with post-treatment (8 or 12 weeks) rates of 0% to 1.4%[66,67,68] and a 1 year follow-up rate of 4% (both treatment groups).[67,68] Allergic reactions to treatment were reported in 3 studies with no differences between silver cream and standard care,[38] silver cream and copper cream,[63] or silver cream and non-adherent dressing.[64] One study reported no treatment-related adverse events associated with a silver or non-silver foam dressing.[65]

Intermittent Pneumatic Compression Therapy

One fair quality RCT followed 54 patients over 26 weeks comparing intermittent pneumatic compression (IPC) therapy to compression bandaging (Unna's boot).[69] Ulcer location was not reported and the trial did not include a run-in period. The mean age of the participants was 57 years; 46% were male. Mean ulcer area was 9.9 cm^2 and mean ulcer duration was 44 weeks. Patients with an ABI of less than 0.9 were excluded; no information was provided about infection status or antibiotic use. The study reported no significant differences between treatment arms in ulcer size or ulcer duration but there were gender differences. In addition to IPC treatment (HRx, Kendall Healthcare Products Co., Mansfield MA) twice a day for 3 hours total, patients in the IPC group wore a HomeRx Therapeutic (Kendall) below-knee gradient compression elastic stocking. It was reported that 93% complied with therapy. Demographic and ulcer characteristics are reported in Appendix D, Table 1.

Primary Outcomes (Appendix D, Table 2)

There was no significant difference between IPC therapy and Unna's boot in percentage of ulcers healed (71% versus 60%, p=ns).[69] It was noted that 100% of ulcers less than 3 cm^2 healed regardless of the treatment group.

Secondary Outcomes (Appendix D, Tables 3, 4, and 5)

Pain ratings on a visual analog scale (VAS) did not differ between intermittent pneumatic compression and compression bandaging.[69] There were no significant differences between treatment groups in the percentage of withdrawals due to adverse events or the percentage of patients having an allergic reaction to treatment.

Electromagnetic Therapy

Two RCTs evaluated electromagnetic therapy (EMT) compared to sham for the treatment of ulcers due to venous insufficiency.[70,71] Both studies included "leg" ulcers with no further detail on ulcer location. One study was conducted in the UK[71] and one in Italy.[70] Neither study included a run-in period with standard care. One study reported that patients with arterial occlusive disease were excluded. This study also prohibited standard compression therapy and monitored use of EMT by a clock built into the device.[70] Neither study reported inclusion or exclusion criteria for infection. A total of 63 patients, 32 receiving EMT and 31 receiving control were enrolled. The overall mean age in one study was 71 years with a significant difference ($p<0.05$) in age between groups (EMT 600 Hz mean age=59; EMT 600 Hz mean age=78; control mean age=71).[71] The mean age in the second study was 66 years and two-thirds of the patients were female.[70] Comorbidities were not uniformly reported (see Appendix D Table 1). Information about ulcer size and duration is presented in Table 16 (below). In one trial, mean ulcer duration was significantly longer in the placebo group than in the two active treatment groups.[71] Patients in both trials had to have had unsatisfactorily healing venous ulcers of at least 4 weeks duration. The aggregate study quality of the included trials was fair. Funding for one study was provided by industry;[71] the funding source for the second trial was not reported.[70]

EMT in one trial was applied with a single pulse of electrical current generating a magnetic field of 2.8 micro Teslas (mT) at a frequency of 75 Hz with an impulse width of 1.3 ms over 3 to 4 hours a day up to 90 days or until the ulcer healed.[70] No compression therapy was administered during the study. In the second trial, there were two treatment arms of EMT, 600 Hz and a magnetic field of 25 mT, and 800 Hz and a magnetic field of 25 mT.[71] Treatments were delivered 5 days a week for 30 days followed by a month of observation.

Table 16. Ulcer Size, Ulcer Duration, and Definitions of Closure: Electromagnetic Therapy

Study / Location	Mean ulcer size, (range or SD)	Duration of ulcer, (range)	Definition of ulcer closure
Kenkre 1996 / UK[71]	EMT 600 Hz: 63 mg (6 to 269) EMT 800 Hz: 81 mg (46 to 197) Control: 119 mg (35 to 526)	EMT 600 Hz: 230.4 weeks (36 to 728) EMT 800 Hz: 418 weeks (36 to 1368) Control: 962.6 weeks (160 to 2548)	NR
Ieran 1990 / Italy[70]	EMT: <15 cm² 4.8, >15 cm² 34.2 Control: <15 cm² 5.0, >15 cm² 39.9	EMT: 30 months (3 to 360) Control: 23 months (3 to 240)	Complete epithelialization

Primary Outcomes (Appendix D, Table 2)

Due to variations in follow-up durations the trials were not statistically pooled. Individual trial risk ratios are presented in Figure 11. The longer-term trial reported a statistically significant difference in healed ulcers in favor of EMT therapy.[70] At day 90, 67% of patients in the EMT group had healed venous ulcers versus 32% of patients in the sham control group arm (ARD=35%, 95% CI 5% to 65%; RR=2.11, 95% CI 1.01 to 4.42).[70] At one-year following the initiation of treatment, 16 patients (89%) in the EMT had healed ulcers compared to 8 patients (42%) in the sham control arm (RR=2.11, 95% CI 1.22 to 3.67). In the second trial, at 50 days from initiation of therapy, 20% of the patients in the combined EMT groups had healed venous ulcers compared to 22% of the patients in the sham control group (RR=0.90, 95% CI 0.16 to 5.13).[71]

Figure 11. Proportion of ulcers healed – Electromagnetic Therapy versus Sham

Study or Subgroup	EMT Events	Total	Control Events	Total	Risk Ratio M-H, Random, 95% CI	Risk Ratio M-H, Random, 95% CI
2.1.1 EMT versus sham (90 days)						
Ieran 1990	12	18	6	19	2.11 [1.01, 4.42]	
2.1.2 EMT versus sham (50 days)						
Kenkre 1996	2	10	2	9	0.90 [0.16, 5.13]	

```
        0.2    0.5    1      2      5
          Favors EMT  Favors control
```

One trial reported average times to healing of 76 days in the EMT group and 71 days in the sham control group but the significance of this difference was not reported.[70] Effectiveness of treatment was also reported. Based on assessment by three physicians blinded to treatment, 15 patients in the EMT group were rated as "excellent" (n=5), or "good" (n=10) compared to 10 patients in the sham control group (2 and 8, respectively). Four patients in the control group and no EMT patients had ulcers rated as "bad" (worsening) (p=0.02). The percentage of patients considered "not restricted" in activity did not differ significantly between the EMT and sham groups.[70] The second trial also reported on activity level. Patients in the 800 Hz and sham control groups improved in their ability to walk up a flight of stairs following treatment.[71] All treatment arms improved in walking a distance consistent with a block of houses and frequency of participating in social activities.

Secondary Outcomes (Appendix D, Tables 3, 4, and 5)

One study reported ulcer recurrence.[70] At follow-up of one year or greater after healing, ulcers recurred in 4 EMT patients and 4 sham control patients. The proportion of healed ulcers after at least one year of follow-up from time of healing was 67% in the EMT group (12 patients) and 21% in the sham control group (4 patients) (RR=3.17, 95% CI 1.25 to 8.03). Both studies reported ulcers infected during treatment. In one study, at day 90, infected ulcers were reported in 3 EMT and 11 control patients.[70] In the other study, no EMT patients and 2 control group patients had infected ulcers.[71] Both studies also reported pain scores. In one study, there was no significant difference between the groups in the amount of pain reported at day 90.[70] In the other study, there were significant reductions (p<0.05) in pain scores from baseline to day 30 for both EMT groups with a non-significant reduction in the control group. The reductions in pain scores in the EMT groups were significantly greater than the reduction in the control group.[71] In one trial, 68% (13/19) of all patients were reported to have experienced adverse events, none leading to study withdrawal.[71] These included moderate-to-severe headaches (2 EMT patients) and sensations of heat, tingling, and "needles and pins" in the limbs (3 patients in each group). Adverse events were not reported in the second trial but 2 of 7 patients not included in the analyses (both in the EMT group) were withdrawn from the study, one after suffering an allergic reaction to medications and one after being diagnosed with rheumatoid arthritis.[70] One study reported no deaths;[70] the second reported no deaths in the EMT group.[71]

Hyberbaric Oxygen

We identified one small double-blinded trial evaluating HBOT for the treatment of venous leg ulcers.[72] Patients were allocated to either HBOT or air at 2.5 ATA for 90 minutes for five days a week for a total of 30 treatments over 6 weeks. The authors reported 100% compliance with the treatment sessions. Patients also continued their pre-study treatment regimen. The trial of 16 patients was conducted in Sweden and included eight men and eight women. Infection status at baseline was not reported. All patients had "normal" ABI values. The median age was 67 years (range 42 to 75). All patients had chronic (greater than 1 year duration), non-diabetic ulcers that ranged from 20.9 to 307.0 cm^2 in size in the HBOT group (8 patients) and 22.1 to 196.9 cm^2 in size in the sham (air) group (8 patients). The trial satisfactorily met the four study quality domains and was therefore considered good quality. Study details are presented in Appendix D, Table 1.

Primary Outcomes (Appendix D, Table 2)

No ulcers were reported healed at post-treatment (week 6). Within 12 weeks after the post-treatment assessment (i.e., week 18), two patients (25%) in the HBOT group had healed ulcers and none in the sham group. Five patients were not available for evaluation at this time-point, three in the sham group and two in the HBOT group. Both of the healed ulcers were initially among the smallest, measuring less than 40 cm^2 at baseline. No definition of healing was provided.[72]

Secondary Outcomes (Appendix D, Tables 3, 4, and 5)

No secondary outcomes were reported.

Summary of Key Question 2

We identified 20 trials of nine different advanced ulcer care therapies for patients with venous ulcers: collagen, biological dressings, biological skin equivalents, keratinocytes, platelet-rich plasma, silver products, intermittent pneumatic compression therapy, electromagnetic therapy, and hyperbaric oxygen therapy. Sixteen of twenty studies compared an advanced therapy to standard therapy.

Primary Outcomes

For collagen, platelet-rich plasma, intermittent pneumatic compression therapy, and hyperbaric oxygen therapy, no eligible studies reported a significant improvement in the number of ulcers healed. Strength of evidence was low for each of those comparisons with only one trial for each advanced wound care therapy (see Executive Summary Table 2). For biological dressings, we found low strength of evidence of improved healing compared with standard care (55% versus 34% healed). The biological skin equivalent Apligraf significantly increased healed ulcers compared to compression bandaging in one trial (63% versus 49%) but the strength of evidence was low. In two trials, Dermagraft was not significantly better than compression bandaging. One trial comparing a keratinocyte product to standard care found improved healing versus standard care although a second trial found no difference. The pooled risk ratio was significant with healing in 38% versus 24% (RR=1.57, 95% CI 1.16-2.11; p=0.003). Two trials of keratinocyte therapies found no difference in ulcer healing when compared to another advanced wound care therapy. Silver creams improved healing in two studies (one comparing silver cream to standard care and one comparing silver cream to a copper-based cream) while three studies of silver dressings found mixed results (significant benefit in one study of silver dressing compared to non-silver dressing and no differences in two studies with non-silver or alternative silver dressings as the comparator). Strength of evidence was low for these outcomes. Two trials of electromagnetic therapy found mixed results; strength of evidence was low.

Few studies reported time to ulcer healing. Two studies of the biological skin equivalent Apligraf found shorter time to ulcer healing as did the study comparing a keratinocyte product to standard care. Two other keratinocyte studies reported no significant differences in time to ulcer healing as did a study comparing a silver dressing to a non-silver dressing. Strength of evidence was low for these comparisons. Two studies of silver products reported higher global assessment outcomes in the silver groups; a study of electromagnetic therapy reported no difference between groups. Only studies of electromagnetic therapy reported patient activity levels; one finding no difference between treatment groups and one noting improvements pre- to post-treatment.

Secondary Outcomes

The most commonly reported secondary outcomes were ulcers infected during treatment (8 studies), ulcer recurrence (7 studies), and pain (9 studies). The collagen treatment study reported fewer ulcers infected in the collagen group. No other study reported a difference between treatment groups. The biological dressings study reported fewer recurring ulcers in the active treatment group compared to standard care. No other differences were reported. One of the EMT studies reported a significant reduction in pain from baseline to 30 days in patients receiving EMT. Other studies reporting pain found no differences between treatment groups. No studies reported amputation, revascularization or other surgery, time to recurrence, or need for home care. Two studies reported hospitalization and one reported quality of life with no difference between treatment arms in the studies. No significant differences were observed in all-cause mortality, study withdrawals due to adverse events, or allergic reactions to treatment.

Table 17. Strength of Evidence – Advanced Wound Care Therapies for Venous Ulcers

Treatment	Control(s)	Outcome	Number of Studies (n for Primary Outcome)*	Comments	Strength of Evidence
Collagen	Standard care	Percentage of ulcers healed	1 (73)	One fair quality RCT found no significant differences between treatment groups.	Low
		Mean time to ulcer healing		Outcome not reported.	Insufficient
Biological Dressings	Standard care with compression bandage	Percentage of ulcers healed	1 (120)	One fair quality study found biological dressing (OASIS) more effective at 12 weeks but not 6 months versus standard care.	Low
		Mean time to ulcer healing		Outcome not reported.	Insufficient
Biological Skin Equivalents [BSE] - *Dermagraft*	Standard care with compression bandage	Percentage of ulcers healed	2 (44)	Data from two small trials (fair quality) found *Dermagraft* was not more effective than standard care.	Low
		Mean time to ulcer healing		Outcome not reported.	Insufficient
Biological Skin Equivalents [BSE] - *Apligraf*	Standard care with compression bandage	Percentage of ulcers healed	1 (275)	One large fair quality trial found significant improvement with *Apligraf* versus standard compression therapy.	Low
		Mean time to ulcer healing		Significant improvement with *Apligraf* versus standard compression therapy.	Low
Keratinocyte Therapy	Standard care with compression bandage	Percentage of ulcers healed	2 (418)	Keratinocyte therapy was more effective than standard care (RR=1.57, 95% CI 1.16 to 2.11, I^2=0%). The trials were rated fair quality.	Moderate
		Mean time to ulcer healing		Inconsistent results, one trial found a significant difference versus standard care and one found no difference between groups.	Low
Keratinocyte Therapy (*Cryopreserved*)	Advanced therapy control (*Lyophilized keratinocytes*)	Percentage of ulcers healed	1 (50)	One poor quality trial reported no differences between treatment groups.	Low
		Mean time to ulcer healing		No difference between groups.	Low
Keratinocyte Therapy	Advanced therapy control (*Pneumatic compression*)	Percentage of ulcers healed	1 (27)	One fair quality trial reported no differences between treatment groups.	Low
		Mean time to ulcer healing		Outcome not reported.	Insufficient
Platelet-Rich Plasma	Placebo	Percentage of ulcers healed	1 (86)	One fair quality trial reported no differences between treatment groups.	Low
		Mean time to ulcer healing		Outcome not reported.	Insufficient

Advanced Wound Care Therapies for Non-Healing Diabetic, Venous, and Arterial Ulcers: A Systematic Review

Treatment	Control(s)	Outcome	Number of Studies (n for Primary Outcome)*	Comments	Strength of Evidence
Silver, Dressings	Controls (non-silver dressing, ionic silver vs. lipido-colloid silver)	Percentage of ulcers healed	3 (536)	Inconsistent results from two fair quality trials, one found a significant difference versus non-silver dressing and one found no difference. One fair quality trial found no difference between two silver dressing groups.	Low
		Mean time to ulcer healing	2 (250)	Two fair quality trials; one found no significant difference between silver and non-silver dressings; one did not report significance	Low
Silver, Cream/ Ointment	Controls (placebo, non-adherent dressing, standard care)	Percentage of ulcers healed	3 (199)	One fair quality trial found significant benefit compared to standard care; one fair and one good quality trail found no benefit compared to placebo or standard dressing	Low
		Mean time to ulcer healing		Outcome not reported.	Insufficient
Silver, Cream	Placebo, tri-peptide copper cream	Percentage of ulcers healed	1 (86)	One three-armed trial of fair quality trial found silver more effective than tri-peptide copper cream but not placebo.	Low
		Mean time to ulcer healing		Outcome not reported.	Insufficient
Intermittent Pneumatic Compression (IPC)	Unna's boot dressing	Percentage of ulcers healed	1 (53)	One fair quality trial found no significant difference between groups.	Low
		Mean time to ulcer healing		Outcome not reported.	Insufficient
Electromagnetic Therapy (EMT)	Sham	Percentage of ulcers healed	2 (56)	Inconsistent results between trials. Study quality was fair.	Low
		Mean time to ulcer healing	1 (37)	Comparable between groups.	Low
Hyperbaric Oxygen Therapy (HBOT)	Sham	Percentage of ulcers healed	1 (16)	One good quality trial found no significant difference between groups.	Low
		Mean time to ulcer healing		Outcome not reported.	Insufficient

*Number of ulcers evaluated for the primary outcome.

The evidence is rated using the following grades: (1) high strength indicates further research is very unlikely to change the confidence in the estimate of effect, meaning that the evidence reflects the true effect; (2) moderate strength denotes further research may change our confidence in the estimate of effect and may change the estimate; (3) low strength indicates further research is very likely to have an important impact on the confidence in the estimate of effect and is likely to change the estimate, meaning there is low confidence that the evidence reflects the true effect; and (4) insufficient, indicating that the evidence is unavailable or does not permit a conclusion.

KEY QUESTION #3. What are the efficacy and harms of therapies for arterial ulcers? Is efficacy dependent on ancillary therapies? Does efficacy differ according to patient demographics, comorbid conditions, treatment compliance, or activity level?

Overview of Studies

We identified one trial of advanced wound care for ulcers attributed to arterial insufficiency,[73] seven trials of advance wound care for lower extremity ulcers of mixed etiology,[74-80] and one trial of advanced wound care for amputation ulcers[81,82] (Table 18).

The study of arterial ulcers compared a biological skin equivalent to standard care. Forty-eight percent of the included ulcers were located on the forefoot, 7% were located on the heel, and 45% were partial open foot amputations (transmetatarsal level).

The studies of mixed ulcer etiologies included 3 studies of biological dressings, 3 studies of silver products, and 1 trial of negative pressure wound therapy. The ulcers were described only as leg ulcers in 4 studies. One study included lower leg extremity ulcers (foot and ankle). In one study, 97% of the ulcers were located on the lower leg and 3% on the ankle or foot.

The trial of amputation ulcers compared negative pressure wound therapy to standard care in patients with partial foot amputation wounds.

No trials of collagen, keratinocytes, platelet-derived growth factors, platelet-rich plasma, pneumatic compression therapy, electromagnetic therapy, hyperbaric oxygen therapy, topical oxygen therapy, or ozone-oxygen therapy were identified that addressed Key Question #3.

Arterial Ulcers

Biological Skin Equivalent

We identified a single RCT of 31 patients that evaluated the use of Apligraf in arterial ulcers following revascularization surgery.[73] This study, based in the United States, was of fair quality. The source of funding was not reported. The mean age of the study participants was 70 years and 77% were male. Race/ethnicity was not reported. All study ulcers were 2.0 cm^2 or larger with an average ulcer size of 4.8 cm^2 at baseline. Ulcer duration was not reported. Participants were patients with ischemic ulcers who had successfully undergone revascularization surgery (ABI <0.5 pre-surgery, >0.7 post-surgery) within 60 days of entering the trial. Patients were followed until ulcer closure or up to 6 months after randomization. A single application of Apligraf was used in 21 patients (10 had a meshed graft and 11 had unmeshed graft) and was compared to 10 patients receiving twice-daily moist dressing changes (considered standard care). Additional study information is presented in Appendix D, Table 1.

Primary Outcomes (Appendix D, Table 2)

Statistically significant improvements in the incidence of complete ulcer healing were seen for the Apligraf group at weeks 8, 12, and 24. At 12 weeks, 86% of Apligraf patients and 40% of control patients had completely healed (p<0.01). At 6 months, complete healing occurred

75

in 100% of the Apligraf group and 75% of the controls. A significant benefit in median time to closure was also seen for Apligraf (7 weeks versus 15 weeks for standard care, p=0.002).[73] Patients in the treatment group also received continuous Unna boot dressing changes until the skin equivalent graft matured (around 5 weeks, on average). As there was no internal control for the additional dressing, more frequent ulcer checks, and recommendation for off-loading in the treatment group, the effect of ancillary therapies could not be measured.

Table 18. Overview of Therapies for Arterial Ulcers, Mixed Lower Extremity Ulcers, and Amputation Wounds

Study, year	N Randomized	Treatment	Product	Comparator	Healed ulcers	Mean time to ulcer healing	Global assessment	Return to daily activities	Ulcers infected during treatment	Amputation	Revascularization/ surgery	Recurrence	Time to Recurrence	Pain/discomfort	Hospitalization	Required home care	Quality of life	Withdrawals due to adverse events	Patients with ≥ 1 adverse event	All-cause mortality	Allergic reactions to treatment
Arterial Ulcers																					
Chang 2000[73]	31	BSE	Apligraf	Standard	+	+			-			-						-	-	-	
Mixed Lower Extremity Ulcers																					
Brigido 2006[74]	28	Col	Graftjacket	Sharp debridement + Curasol gel	+	±													-		
Romanelli 2007[75]	54	BD	OASIS	Hyaluronic acid dressing	+				-					+				-	-	-	
Romanelli 2010[76]	50	BD	OASIS	Standard	+	+			-					-				-	-	-	
Jørgensen 2005[77]	129	Silver foam dressing	Contreet	Non-silver foam dressing	-									-			-		-		
Miller 2010[78]	281	Silver dressing	Multiple products	Cadexomer iodine dressing	-	-													-		
Fumal 2002[79]	17	Silver cream		Standard	-	-															
Vuerstaek 2006[80]	60	NPWT	V.A.C	Standard	-	+			-	-		-	-	+/-	-			-	-	-	
Amputation Wounds																					
Armstrong 2005, Apelqvist 2008[81,82]	162	NPWT	V.A.C.	Standard	+	+			→						-				-		

BD – Biological Dressing; BSE – Biological Skin Equivalent; Col – Collagen; NPWT – Negative Pressure Wound Therapy
+ Treatment group better than comparator (p< 0.05)
- Treatment group demonstrated no significant benefit
→ Treatment group worse than comparator
± Significance could not be determined

Secondary Outcomes (Appendix D, Tables 3, 4, and 5)

Three localized, indolent ulcer infections were reported in the Apligraf group with no infections in the control group. The difference between groups was not significant. There was also no difference between treatment groups in ulcer recurrence. No differences between groups were reported for adverse events, withdrawals due to adverse events, or all-cause mortality.[73]

Studies of Mixed Ulcer Types

Collagen

One fair quality trial (n=28) compared a collagen product (Graftjacket) to standard care.[74] Study characteristics and outcomes data are reported in Appendix D, Tables 1 to 5. The mean age of the patients was 64 years. Gender, ulcer size, and ulcer duration were not provided but it was reported that patient age and ulcer size were similar for the two treatment groups at baseline. Patients were required to have a palpable/audible pulse in the affected lower extremity; patients with infected ulcers were excluded. Standard care included off-loading but compliance was not reported. A significantly higher percentage of healed ulcers was found in the Graftjacket group compared to standard care (86% versus 29%, p=0.01). No difference was observed in mean time to ulcer healing. Number of ulcers infected during treatment and number of patients experiencing adverse events also did not differ between the collagen and standard care groups.

Biological Dressings

Two randomized controlled trials evaluated biological dressings (OASIS) in patients with mixed (arterial or venous) or non-specific chronic lower-extremity ulcers.[75,76] One study comparing a biological dressing with another advanced therapy (hyaluronic acid dressing) was of poor quality[75] and one study comparing a biological dressing with standard care was of fair quality.[76] Neither study included a run-in period with standard care or reported on compliance with therapy or antibiotic use. Both trials excluded patients with infected wounds and ABI less than 0.6. One study reported mean age (63 years);[75] in both studies 48% of the patients were male. Mean ulcer size was 6 cm² in one study[75] and 24.4 cm² in the other.[76] Mean ulcer durations were similar (7.8 and 7.1 weeks). The studies reported no differences between treatment arms at baseline. Study characteristics and outcomes data are presented in Appendix D, Tables 1 to 5.

Both studies reported a significantly higher percentage of ulcers healed by study completion for the biological dressing compared to either another advanced wound therapy (81% versus 46%, p<0.001)[75] or standard care (80% versus 65%, p<0.05).[76] One study reported time to complete ulcer healing finding a significantly shorter mean time to ulcer healing with biological dressing compared to standard care (5.4 weeks versus 8.3 weeks, p=0.02).[76] One study reported no difference between a biological dressing and standard care in ulcers infected during treatment.[76] Both studies reported on pain. One found a significant reduction in pain in the biological dressing group compared to another advanced wound therapy;[75] the second reported no difference between biological dressing and standard care.[76] No significant differences in withdrawals due to adverse events, patients experiencing adverse events, or all-cause mortality were observed (no events in either treatment group in either study).

Silver Products

Three fair quality studies reported on the use of silver products for patients with mixed ulcer types. One study included 129 patients with chronic venous or mixed venous/arterial ulcers of at least 2 cm^2 (with no decrease in area of greater than 0.5 cm in the past 4 weeks), ABI of 0.65 or higher, and signs of infection.[77] Median age was 74 years and 36% of the patients were male. Median ulcer size was 6.4 cm^2 and median ulcer duration was 1.1 years. Patients were treated with a silver-releasing foam dressing or a similar dressing without silver. The second study included 281 patients with venous and mixed ulcers with a diameter of 15 cm or less.[78] All patients had clinical signs of infection and an ABI of 0.6 or higher; patients with a diagnosis of diabetes were excluded. Approximately 20% of the patients required antibiotics. Seventy-four percent of the ulcers were venous. One group received a silver-based dressing and the other group received an iodine-based dressing. Compression bandaging was part of the treatment for both groups and compliance with compression was monitored. Mean age of the participants was 80 years with 41% male. The mean ulcer size was 705 mm^2 and mean ulcer duration was 54 weeks. There was a significant difference in baseline ulcer size between the silver dressing group (597 mm^2) and the iodine dressing group (912 mm^2). The third study enrolled 17 patients with at least 2 chronic leg ulcers.[79] Patients with infection, diabetes, or arterial occlusion were excluded. Mean age of the participants was 55 years; other baseline characteristics were not reported. Two similar looking ulcers on each patient were randomly assigned to treatment with silver sulfadiazine cream or standard care for 6 weeks.

The two studies reporting healed ulcers found no significant difference between a silver-releasing foam dressing and a similar dressing without silver (9.6% versus 8.8% at 4 weeks)[77] or a silver dressing and an iodine dressing (64% versus 63% at 12 weeks).[78] The study comparing silver and iodine dressings also reported no significant difference in days to healing.[78] The third study did not report healed ulcers but did report a non-significant difference in time to healing (15 weeks for silver-treated ulcers, 16 weeks for standard care).[79] One study looked at subgroups.[78] There was no difference in number of ulcers healed with silver or iodine dressings for "young" ulcers (less than 12 weeks), "old" ulcers (more than 12 weeks), "small" ulcers (3.6 cm^2 or smaller), or "large" ulcers (greater than 3.6 cm^2).[78] Decrease in pain during the treatment period and quality of life were found to be similar in patients treated with silver-releasing foam dressing compared to non-silver foam dressing.[77] Two studies reported adverse events. The percentages of patients with adverse events (silver dressing versus iodine dressing)[78] or device-related adverse events(silver-releasing foam dressing versus non-silver foam dressing)[77] did not differ. Additional information about these studies is presented in Appendix D, Tables 1 to 5.

Negative Pressure Wound Therapy

One study of NPWT compared to standard care included venous ulcers (43%), mixed venous and arterial ulcers (13%), and microangiopathic ulcers (43%).[80] The study was of fair quality. Patients with infected ulcers or an ABI of less than 0.6 were excluded. The median age of the participants was 72 years, 23% were male, the median ulcer surface area was 38 cm^2, and the median ulcer duration was 7.5 months. Although not significant, mean ulcer area differed between groups by 10 cm^2 at baseline. Patients were hospitalized for chronic leg ulcers at the time of enrollment and remained hospitalized until complete healing. They were mobile for hygiene only. Antibiotics were allowed as needed (approximately 3.5% of patients at baseline). Patients in the NPWT group received treatment (125 mmHg permanent negative pressure) until granulation tissue covered 100% of the surface and secretion was minimal. They then underwent skin graft transplantation, 4 days of negative pressure therapy, and standard ulcer care until complete healing. The standard care group was treated with either hydrogel or alginate dressings and compression bandage therapy until granulation followed by skin graft transplantation and additional compression therapy.

Complete healing occurred in 96% of patients in both the NPWT and standard care groups. The time to complete healing was shorter in the NPWT group (median of 29 days versus 45 days in the standard care group, p=0.0001). After adjustment for ulcer area, smoking, baseline infection signs, history of ulcers, use of angiotensin-converting enzyme inhibitors, and use of anticlotting therapy, the time to healing remained significantly shorter in the NPTW group than in the standard care group (HR=3.2, 95% CI 1.7 to 6.2, p<0.001). Time to preparation of the ulcer for skin graft transplantation was also shorter in the NPTW group (median of 7 days versus 17 days in the standard care group, p=0.005) and remained shorter after adjustment for baseline factors (HR=2.4, 95% CI 1.2 to 4.7, p<0.01). Ulcer recurrence was similar between the groups (52% NPWT, 42% standard care) but skin graft survival was significantly better in the NPWT group (83% versus 70%, p=0.01). Quality of life scores increased over time with no differences between groups. Pain scores decreased over time and at week 5 and beyond, were significantly lower in the NPWT group. Most ulcers in the NPWT group were healed by that point. There were no differences between NPWT and standard care in infection, mortality, percentage of patient who experienced an adverse event, or percentage of patients who reported pain as an adverse event. More detailed study characteristics and outcomes are presented in Appendix D, Tables 1 to 5.

Amputation Wounds

We identified one good quality study that compared NPWT to standard wound therapy in 162 patients with partial diabetic foot amputation wounds.[81,82] Patients with severely infected wounds or inadequate blood supply were excluded. Standard care included off-loading, as needed; compliance was not reported. The mean age of the patients was 59 years and 81% were male. The mean wound size was 20.7 cm^2 and mean duration was 1.5 months. The percentage of healed wounds (56% versus 39%, p=0.04) was higher and the time to healing was shorter (median days: 56 versus 77, p=0.005) in the NPWT group compared to standard care. A second amputation was required by 3% of the NPWT group and 11% of the standard care group (RR=0.23, 95% CI 0.05 to 1.1, p=0.06). Adverse events were reported for 52% of the NPWT group and 54% of the standard care group (p=0.88) with infections most common (17% in the NPWT group, 6% in the standard care group, p=0.04).[81] An analysis of resource utilization among patients in the study who were treated for a minimum of 8 weeks (n=135) found similar hospital stays with means of 10.6 and 9.9 inpatient days in the NPWT and standard care groups, respectively. The overall number of procedures performed (e.g., debridement, dressing changes, grafts) was significantly higher in the standard care group (mean of 120 procedures versus 43 in the NPWT group, p<0.001). There were also significantly more outpatient visits in the standard care group (mean of 11 visits versus 4 in the NPWT group, p<0.05).[82] Appendix D, Tables 1 to 5 contain more details about the study.

Summary of Key Question 3

For arterial ulcers, one small, fair quality study found that a biological skin equivalent, may improve the incidence and rate of complete ulcer healing when used on ischemic foot ulcers following revascularization surgery. Other outcomes did not differ significantly from standard care. The effects of ancillary therapies or baseline patient characteristics were not explored in the study. We found no RCTs that included any of the other therapies of interest exclusively in patients with arterial lower extremity ulcers.

In seven studies of mixed ulcer types, collagen and biological dressings were found to improve ulcer healing; silver products and negative pressure wound therapy did not. There were mixed results for time to ulcer healing and, overall, no differences between investigational treatment and control on other outcomes. The studies were of poor to fair quality.

One good quality study of ulcers associated with partial foot amputation showed a benefit of NPWT with respect to healed ulcers and mean time to healing. There were significantly more infections in the NPWT group but the incidence of other adverse events did not differ between the NPWT and standard care groups.

SUMMARY AND DISCUSSION

Chronic lower extremity ulcers are a common and serious health problem. A wide range of standard treatment approaches to achieve ulcer healing are used (e.g., off-loading, compression, leg elevation etc.) based on patient and ulcer factors and provider preferences. While many ulcers heal completely within several weeks, a significant portion either do not heal or increase in size, depth, and severity. These chronic ulcers can result in considerable clinical morbidity and health care costs.

Many types of advanced wound care therapies exist but all represent considerably greater product costs compared to standard therapy. These costs may be justified if they result in improved ulcer healing, reduced morbidity, fewer lower extremity amputations, and improved patient functional status. In addition to the treatment selected, many potential factors contribute to the success or failure of the ulcer healing process including ulcer etiology; ulcer area, depth, duration, and location; patient comorbid conditions; and patient compliance with the treatment protocol. Much of the existing research on advanced wound care therapies has attempted to minimize the influence of many of these factors by limiting enrollment to patients with ulcers of a particular size, including only patients with adequate circulation, and excluding patients taking certain classes of medications.[83,84] Furthermore, many of the trials are industry sponsored (55% of the studies included in our review) and the role of the sponsor is typically not stated, definitions of "chronic" ulcers vary widely, and few studies are of sufficient duration to assess whether healing is maintained.[84,85]

Our systematic review of randomized controlled trials found discouragingly low strength evidence regarding the effectiveness and comparative effectiveness of advanced wound care therapies for treatment of lower extremity ulcers. This was primarily due to the fact that for each ulcer type (diabetic, venous, or arterial) individual categories of advanced wound care therapies were only evaluated in a few studies, often in highly selected populations, and frequently had conflicting findings. Furthermore, within each category of wound care therapies several different types of interventions were used making it difficult to determine if results were replicable in other studies or generalizable to broader clinical settings. Additionally, most studies compared advanced wound care therapies to standard care or placebo. Therefore there is little comparative effectiveness research evaluating one advanced wound care therapy to another. It has been noted that standard care is an inappropriate comparator for studies of advanced therapy since patients have likely already failed standard care.[86,87] For arterial ulcers we identified only a single study of any advanced wound care therapy (and this was compared to standard care) despite the clinical importance of arterial ulcers.

However, based on the available findings we conclude that for patients with diabetic chronic ulcers, there is moderate strength of evidence that the biological skin equivalent Apligraf and negative pressure wound therapy improve healing compared to standard care. There is low strength evidence that advanced wound care therapies improved the percentage of ulcers healed compared to standard care for the following therapies: collagen (notably Graftjacket), the biological skin equivalent Dermagraft, platelet-derived growth factors, silver cream, and hyperbaric oxygen therapy but results were not uniform for any treatment group. Most beneficial effects were derived from single or few studies so we recommend caution regarding translating these findings of effectiveness into broader clinical application. Pooled analyses were possible for several therapies and demonstrated a significant improvement in ulcer healing compared to standard care for Apligraf (a biological skin equivalent), platelet-derived growth factors, and negative pressure wound therapy; no improvement was observed for Dermagraft (a biological skin equivalent). Few studies compared one advanced treatment to another but in those studies, no differences in percentage of ulcers healed were found between the two treatment arms. For time to ulcer healing, the pattern of findings was similar and strength of evidence was low for all treatment comparisons reporting that outcome. No studies reported a significant difference in adverse events for any treatment comparison.

Findings for venous ulcers were similar. Although some individual trials of biological dressings (notably OASIS), biological skin equivalents (Apligraf), keratinocytes, silver cream and dressing, and electromagnetic therapy noted significant benefit of the therapy in percentage of ulcers healed compared to standard care, overall the results for each therapy were mixed. In pooled analyses only keratinocytes resulted in significantly better healing compared to standard care. Strength of evidence was moderate for the benefit of keratinocyte therapy and low for the other therapies. Few studies of venous ulcers compared two advanced therapies and, where reported, typically found no differences. Time to ulcer healing was reported infrequently. No advanced wound care therapy was observed to result in an increase in adverse events.

We identified only one study of patients with arterial ulcers despite the clinical importance of this population. It is possible that patients with arterial disease were included in the studies of diabetic ulcers or venous ulcers (i.e., mixed etiology). In one study of patients with non-healing lower extremity ulcers or amputation wounds following a revascularization procedure, Apligraf increased ulcer healing and decreased time to healing compared to standard care with no difference in adverse events.

For amputation wounds, one study of negative pressure wound therapy versus standard care found significantly better healing with no difference in adverse events.

Despite finding benefits of some therapies compared to standard care, the methodological quality of individual studies reviewed was predominantly fair or poor. Common factors limiting the quality were inadequate allocation concealment, no blinding (including no blinding of outcome assessment), failure to use intention-to-treat analysis methods, and failure to adequately describe study dropouts and withdrawals. With methodological flaws, few trials reporting, and heterogeneity in the comparators, study duration, and how outcomes were assessed, the overall strength of evidence was low. While a wide range of patients were enrolled in studies most were older than age 60 years, male, of white race, likely compliant with treatment protocols, and possessed ulcers that were relatively small as measured by surface area. However, authors rarely reported outcomes by patient demographic, comorbidity or ulcer characteristics. Therefore, we found insufficient evidence to guide clinicians and policy makers regarding whether efficacy differs according to patient demographics, comorbid conditions, treatment compliance, or activity level.

APPLICABILITY AND COST EFFECTIVENESS

It is not well known how outcomes reported in studies of selected populations will translate to daily practice settings including in Veterans Health Administration facilities. There is evidence of good success in ulcer healing with strict adherence to off-loading for diabetic ulcers and compression therapy for venous ulcers.[88-91] The patients enrolled in trials were likely more compliant than typical patients and received very close monitoring. Therefore, results from these studies may overestimate benefits and underestimate harms in non-study populations.

Our review was limited to studies of FDA approved products. We excluded studies with wounds of multiple etiologies (e.g., vascular, pressure, trauma, surgery) if they did not report results by etiology. We also excluded studies if they did not report our primary outcomes of healed wounds or time to complete healing. Many studies report change in ulcer size but the clinical benefit of change in ulcer size has not been established.[92]

Furthermore, we did not conduct cost effectiveness analyses or assess additional costs of care associated with chronic ulcers. Despite the high costs of advanced wound care therapies it is possible that they may be cost effective or even cost saving if found to improve ulcer healing; reduce ulcer associated morbidity, hospitalizations, medical care and amputations; and improve functional status and quality of life. Based on our findings from randomized controlled trials the decision of if, when, and in whom to use advanced wound care therapies as well as the type of advanced wound care therapy selected is difficult. Additionally, because little comparative effectiveness research exists to guide choices, decisions may be based on other factors including wound care product cost, ease of use, and patient and provider preferences (the latter also influenced by personal experience with ulcer and patient characteristics).

RECOMMENDATIONS FOR FUTURE RESEARCH

Our review highlights several much needed areas for future research. Most studies compared an advanced therapy to either standard ulcer care or placebo treatment. Few studies (10 of the 35 eligible studies of diabetic ulcers, 4 of the 20 eligible studies of venous ulcers, and none for arterial or mixed ulcers) directly compared two advanced therapies. Furthermore, few studies provided a run-in period with carefully monitored standard care to exclude patients for whom carefully monitored standard care would obviate the need for advanced therapy. Therefore, additional randomized trials of advanced wound care therapies versus standard care are needed to replicate or refute current findings. Comparative effectiveness research is also needed to evaluate the relative benefits and harms of different advanced wound care therapies. In both effectiveness and comparative effectiveness research, the sample sizes should be adequate to report specific outcome reporting according to key patient and ulcer characteristics including age, race, gender, and ulcer size, location, and depth. We note below the limitations of the existing research by type of ulcer and therapy assessed.

Of the studies of diabetic ulcers included in this review, only two focused on biological dressings (using different products) and two on platelet-rich plasma. We identified no studies of topical oxygen or electromagnetic therapy. No studies reported on return to daily activities or the need for home care related to ulcer treatment and only one study reported quality of life or hospitalization. The need for amputation or revascularization and the incidence of and time to ulcer recurrence require further investigation. The majority of studies described the ulcers as diabetic foot ulcers with only six providing greater detail about ulcer location. Future research should report healing by ulcer location. Future research should also examine microvascular disease to more clearly distinguish diabetic ulcers from arterial ulcers.

For venous ulcers, we identified only one study of the following advanced wound care therapies: collagen, biological dressings, platelet rich plasma, intermittent pneumatic compression, and hyperbaric oxygen therapy. There were no studies of platelet-derived growth factors or typical oxygen. We found no studies that reported on amputations, time to ulcer recurrence, or need for home health care related to the ulcer. One study reported hospitalization, one study reported quality of life, and two studies reported return to work or daily activities.

We identified only one study of patients with arterial disease requiring advanced wound care following revascularization. Only this study and one other included patients with partial foot amputations with delayed healing. Neither of these studies reported on return to daily activities, pain, quality of life, or need for home health assistance related to the wound. There is a paucity of research on advanced wound care therapies in patients with strictly arterial disease.

In addition to specific topics needing further research, several organizations have outlined overall methodological standards for future research of wound healing therapies (see Appendix E). The standards focus on study design, patient population, comparators, outcomes and outcome assessment, and potential sources of bias. Randomized trials, with allocation concealment and, at a minimum, blinding of third-party outcomes assessors, are recommended. The patient population should be appropriate for the treatment being studied and exclusion criteria should be minimal to enhance generalizability. Endpoints should be selected based on the purpose of the intervention (i.e., closure versus preparation for surgery) and adequate follow-up should be included to confirm healing. Dropouts and study withdrawals should be documented, including withdrawals due to ulcer deterioration. Additional research, conducted in accordance with the standards, is needed to establish the safety and efficacy of advanced wound care therapies. Finally, future research is needed to determine the effectiveness, comparative effectiveness and harms of advanced wound care therapies as used in general clinical practice settings (e.g., vascular and dermatology clinics) where patients may have more severe and larger ulcers, greater comorbidities, or increased difficulty with treatment compliance.

REFERENCES

1. Sen CK, Gordillo GM, Roy S, et al. Human skin wounds: a major and snowballing threat to public health and the economy. *Wound Repair Regen.* 2009;17(6):763-71.

2. Jones KR, Fennie K, Lenihan A. Evidence-based management of chronic wounds. *Adv Skin Wound Care.* 2007;20(11):591-600.

3. Spentzouris G, Labropoulos N. The evaluation of lower-extremity ulcers. *Semin Intervent Radiol.* 2009;26(4):286-95.

4. Ayello EA. What does the wound say? Why determining etiology is essential for appropriate wound care. *Adv Skin Wound Care.* 2005;18(2):98-109.

5. American Society of Plastic Surgeons. Evidence-based Clinical Practice Guideline: Chronic Wounds of the Lower Extremity. 2007. Available at: http://www.plasticsurgery. org/Documents/medical-professionals/health-policy/evidence-practice/Evidence-based-Clinical-Practice-Guideline-Chronic-Wounds-of-the-Lower-Extremity.pdf. Accessed September 2012.

6. Hess CT. Lower-extremity wound checklist. *Adv Skin Wound Care.* 2011;24(3):144.

7. McCulloch DK, de Asia RJ. Management of diabetic foot lesions. In: Basow DS, ed. UpToDate. Waltham, MA. 2012.

8. Wagner FW, Jr. The dysvascular foot: a system for diagnosis and treatment. *Foot Ankle.* 1981;2(2):64-122.

9. Lavery LA, Armstrong DG, Harkless LB. Classification of diabetic foot wounds. *J Foot Surg.* 1996;35(6):528-31.

10. Valencia IC, Falabella H, Kirsner RS, Eaglstein WH. Chronic venous insufficiency and venous leg ulceration. *J Am Acad Dermatol.* 2001;44:401–21.

11. Nelzen O, Bergqvist D, Lindhagen A. Venous and non-venous leg ulcers: clinical history and appearance in a population study. *Br J Surg.* 1994;81(2):182-7.

12. Mayberry JC, Moneta GL, Taylor LMJr, Porter JM. Fifteen-year results of ambulatory compression therapy for chronic venous ulcers. *Surgery.* 1991;109:575-81.

13. Higgins JPT, Green S (editors). Cochrane Handbook for Systematic Reviews of Interventions Version 5.1.0 [updated March 2011]. The Cochrane Collaboration, 2011. Available from www.cochrane-handbook.org.

14. Owens DK, Lohr KN, Atkins D, et al. AHRQ series paper 5: grading the strength of a body of evidence when comparing medical interventions--agency for healthcare research and quality and the effective health-care program. *J Clin Epidemiol.* 2010 May;63(5):513-23.

15. Blume P, Driver VR, Tallis AJ, et al. Formulated collagen gel accelerates healing rate immediately after application in patients with diabetic neuropathic foot ulcers. *Wound Repair Regen.* 2011;19(3):302-8.

16. Veves A, Sheehan P, Pham HT. A randomized, controlled trial of Promogran (a collagen/oxidized regenerated cellulose dressing) vs standard treatment in the management of diabetic foot ulcers. *Arch Surg.* 2002;137(7):822-7.

17. Donaghue VM, Chrzan JS, Rosenblum BI, Giurini JM, Habershaw GM, Veves A. Evaluation of a collagen-alginate wound dressing in the management of diabetic foot ulcers. *Adv Wound Care.* 1998;11(3):114-9.

18. Reyzelman A, Crews RT, Moore JC, et al. Clinical effectiveness of an acellular dermal regenerative tissue matrix compared to standard wound management in healing diabetic foot ulcers: a prospective, randomised, multicentre study. *Int Wound J.* 2009;6(3):196-208.

19. Niezgoda JA, Van Gils CC, Frykberg RG, Hodde JP. Randomized clinical trial comparing OASIS Wound Matrix to Regranex Gel for diabetic ulcers. *Adv Skin Wound Care.* 2005;18(5 Pt 1):258-66.

20. Landsman A, Roukis TS, DeFronzo DJ, Agnew P, Petranto RD, Surprenant M. Living cells or collagen matrix: which is more beneficial in the treatment of diabetic foot ulcers? *Wounds.* 2008;20(5):111-6.

21. Gentzkow GD, Iwasaki SD, Hershon KS, et al. Use of dermagraft, a cultured human dermis, to treat diabetic foot ulcers. *Diabetes Care.* 1996;19(4):350-4.

22. Naughton G, Mansbridge J, Gentzkow G. A metabolically active human dermal replacement for the treatment of diabetic foot ulcers. *Artif Organs.* 1997;21(11):1203-10.

23. Marston WA, Hanft J, Norwood P, Pollak R, Dermagraft Diabetic Foot Ulcer Study G. The efficacy and safety of Dermagraft in improving the healing of chronic diabetic foot ulcers: results of a prospective randomized trial. *Diabetes Care.* 2003;26(6):1701-5.

24. Veves A, Falanga V, Armstrong DG, Sabolinski ML, Apligraf Diabetic Foot Ulcer S. Graftskin, a human skin equivalent, is effective in the management of noninfected neuropathic diabetic foot ulcers: a prospective randomized multicenter clinical trial. *Diabetes Care.* 2001;24(2):290-5.

25. Edmonds M, European, Australian Apligraf Diabetic Foot Ulcer Study G. Apligraf in the treatment of neuropathic diabetic foot ulcers. *Int J Low Extrem Wounds.* 2009;8(1):11-8.

26. DiDomenico L, Emch KJ, Landsman AR, Landsman A. A prospective comparison of diabetic foot ulcers treated with either a cryopreserved skin allograft or a bioengineered skin substitute. *Wounds.* 2011;23(7):184-9.

27.   Aminian B, Shams M, Soveyd M, Omrani GR. Topical autologous platelet-derived growth factors in the treatment of chronic diabetic ulcers. *Arch Iranian Med.* 2000;3(2):55-9.

28.   Agrawal RP, Jhajharia A, Mohta N, Dogra R, Chaudhari V, Nayak KC. Use of a platelet-derived growth factor gel in chronic diabetic foot ulcers. *Diabetic Foot J.* 2009;12(2):80-8.

29.   Hardikar JV, Reddy YC, Bung DD, et al. Efficacy of recombinant human platelet-derived growth factor (rhPDGF) based gel in diabetic foot ulcers: a randomized, multicenter, double-blind, placebo-controlled study in India. *Wounds.* 2005;17(6):141-52.

30.   Bhansali A, Venkatesh S, Dutta P, Dhillon MS, Das S, Agrawal A. Which is the better option: recombinant human PDGF-BB 0.01% gel or standard wound care, in diabetic neuropathic large plantar ulcers off-loaded by a customized contact cast? *Diabetes Res Clin Pract.* 2009;83(1):e13-16.

31.   Wieman TJ, Smiell JM, Su Y. Efficacy and safety of a topical gel formulation of recombinant human platelet-derived growth factor-BB (becaplermin) in patients with chronic neuropathic diabetic ulcers. A phase III randomized placebo-controlled double-blind study. *Diabetes Care.* 1998;21(5):822-7.

32.   Jaiswal SS, Gambhir RPS, Agrawal A, Harish S. Efficacy of topical recombinant human platelet derived growth factor on wound healing in patients with chronic diabetic lower limb ulcers. *Indian J Surg.* 2010;72(1):31-5.

33.   Steed DL. Clinical evaluation of recombinant human platelet-derived growth factor for the treatment of lower extremity diabetic ulcers. Diabetic Ulcer Study Group. *J Vasc Surg.* 1995;21(1):71-78.

34.   Steed DL. Clinical evaluation of recombinant human platelet-derived growth factor for the treatment of lower extremity ulcers. *Plast Reconstr Surg.* 2006;117 Suppl 7:143-9S.

35.   d'Hemecourt PA, Smiell JM, Karim MR. Sodium carboxymethycellulose aqueous-based gel vs becaplermin gel in patients with nonhealing lower extremity diabetic ulcers. *Wounds.* 1998;10(3):69-75.

36.   Saad Setta H, Elshahat A, Elsherbiny K, Massoud K, Safe I. Platelet-rich plasma versus platelet-poor plasma in the management of chronic diabetic foot ulcers: a comparative study. *Int Wound J.* 2011;8(3):307-12.

37.   Driver VR, Hanft J, Fylling CP, Beriou JM, Autologel Diabetic Foot Ulcer Study G. A prospective, randomized, controlled trial of autologous platelet-rich plasma gel for the treatment of diabetic foot ulcers. *Ostomy Wound Manage.* 2006;52(6):68-70, 74 passim.

38.   Belcaro G, Cesarone MR, Errichi BM, et al. Venous and diabetic ulcerations: management with topical multivalent silver oxide ointment. *Panminerva Med.* 2010;52(2 Suppl 1):37-42.

39.   Jacobs AM, Tomczak R. Evaluation of Bensal HP for the treatment of diabetic foot ulcers. *Adv Skin Wound Care.* 2008;21(10):461-5.

40.   Jude EB, Apelqvist J, Spraul M, Martini J, Silver Dressing Study G. Prospective randomized controlled study of Hydrofiber dressing containing ionic silver or calcium alginate dressings in non-ischaemic diabetic foot ulcers. *Diabet Med.* 2007;24(3):280-8.

41.   Viswanathan V, Kesavan R, Kavitha KV, Kumpatla S. A pilot study on the effects of a polyherbal formulation cream on diabetic foot ulcers. *Indian J Med Res.* 2011;134(2):168-73.

42.   Blume PA, Walters J, Payne W, Ayala J, Lantis J. Comparison of negative pressure wound therapy using vacuum-assisted closure with advanced moist wound therapy in the treatment of diabetic foot ulcers: a multicenter randomized controlled trial. *Diabetes Care.* 2008;31(4):631-6.

43.   Karatepe O, Eken I, Acet E, et al. Vacuum assisted closure improves the quality of life in patients with diabetic foot. *Acta Chir Belg.* 2011;111(5):298-302.

44.   McCallon SK, Knight CA, Valiulus JP, Cunningham MW, McCulloch JM, Farinas LP. Vacuum-assisted closure versus saline-moistened gauze in the healing of postoperative diabetic foot wounds. *Ostomy Wound Manage.* 2000;46(8):28-32, 34.

45.   Wang C-J, Wu R-W, Yang Y-J. Treatment of diabetic foot ulcers: a comparative study of extracorporeal shockwave therapy and hyperbaric oxygen therapy. *Diabetes Res Clin Pract.* 2011;92(2):187-93.

46.   Londahl M, Katzman P, Nilsson A, Hammarlund C. Hyperbaric oxygen therapy facilitates healing of chronic foot ulcers in patients with diabetes. *Diabetes Care.* 2010;33(5):998-1003.

47.   Duzgun AP, Satir HZ, Ozozan O, Saylam B, Kulah B, Coskun F. Effect of hyperbaric oxygen therapy on healing of diabetic foot ulcers. *J Foot Ankle Surg.* 2008;47(6):515-9.

48.   Kessler L, Bilbault P, Ortega F, et al. Hyperbaric oxygenation accelerates the healing rate of nonischemic chronic diabetic foot ulcers: a prospective randomized study. *Diabetes Care.* 2003;26(8):2378-82.

49.   Abidia A, Laden G, Kuhan G, et al. The role of hyperbaric oxygen therapy in ischaemic diabetic lower extremity ulcers: a double-blind randomised-controlled trial. *Eur J Vasc Endovasc Surg.* 2003;25(6):513-8.

50.   Wainstein J, Feldbrin Z, Boaz M, Harman-Boehm I. Efficacy of ozone-oxygen therapy for the treatment of diabetic foot ulcers. *Diabetes Technol Ther.* 2011;13(12):1255-60.

51.   Motzkau M, Tautenhahn J, Lehnert H, Lobmann R. Expression of matrix-metalloproteases in the fluid of chronic diabetic foot wounds treated with a protease absorbent dressing. *Exp Clin Endocrinol.* 2011;119(5):286-90.

52.   Vin F, Teot L, Meaume S. The healing properties of Promogran in venous leg ulcers. *J Wound Care.* 2002;11(9):335-41.

53.   Mostow EN, Haraway GD, Dalsing M, Hodde JP, King D, Group OVUS. Effectiveness of an extracellular matrix graft (OASIS Wound Matrix) in the treatment of chronic leg ulcers: a randomized clinical trial. *J Vasc Surg.* 2005;41(5):837-43.

54.   Falanga V, Margolis D, Alvarez O, et al. Rapid healing of venous ulcers and lack of clinical rejection with an allogeneic cultured human skin equivalent. Human Skin Equivalent Investigators Group. *Arch Dermatol.* 1998;134(3):293-300.

55.   Falanga V, Sabolinski M. A bilayered living skin construct (APLIGRAF) accelerates complete closure of hard-to-heal venous ulcers. *Wound Repair Regen.* 1999;7(4):201-7.

56.   Krishnamoorthy L, Harding K, Griffiths D. The clinical and histological effects of Dermagraft in the healing of chronic venous leg ulcers. *Phlebology.* 2003;18(1):12-22.

57.   Omar AA, Mavor AID, Jones AM, Homer-Vanniasinkam S. Treatment of venous leg ulcers with Dermagraft. *Eur J Vasc Endovasc Surg.* 2004;27(6):666-72.

58.   Lindgren C, Marcusson JA, Toftgard R. Treatment of venous leg ulcers with cryopreserved cultured allogeneic keratinocytes: a prospective open controlled study. *Br J Dermatol.* 1998;139(2):271-5.

59.   Navratilova Z, Slonkova V, Semradova V, Adler J. Cryopreserved and lyophilized cultured epidermal allografts in the treatment of leg ulcers: a pilot study. *J Eur Acad Dermatol Venereol.* 2004;18(2):173-9.

60.   Harding KG, Krieg T, Eming SA, et al. Efficacy and safety of the freeze-dried cultured human keratinocyte lysate, LyphoDerm 0.9%, in the treatment of hard-to-heal venous leg ulcers. *Wound Repair Regen.* 2005;13(2):138-47.

61.   Vanscheidt W, Ukat A, Horak V, et al. Treatment of recalcitrant venous leg ulcers with autologous keratinocytes in fibrin sealant: a multinational randomized controlled clinical trial. *Wound Repair Regen.* 2007;15(3):308-15.

62.   Stacey MC, Mata SD, Trengove NJ, Mather CA. Randomised double-blind placebo controlled trial of topical autologous platelet lysate in venous ulcer healing. *Eur J Vasc Endovasc Surg.* 2000;20(3):296-301.

63.   Bishop JB, Phillips LG, Mustoe TA, et al. A prospective randomized evaluator-blinded trial of two potential wound healing agents for the treatment of venous stasis ulcers. *J Vasc Surg.* 1992;16(2):251-7.

64.   Blair SD, Backhouse CM, Wright DDI, Riddle E, McCollum CN. Do dressings influence the healing of chronic venous ulcers? *Phlebology.* 1988;3:129-34.

65.   Dimakakos E, Katsenis K, Kalemikerakis J, et al. Infected Venous Leg Ulcers: Management With Silver-releasing Foam Dressing. *Wounds.* 2009;21(1):4-8.

66.   Harding K, Gottrup F, Jawien A, et al. A prospective, multi-centre, randomised, open label, parallel, comparative study to evaluate effects of AQUACEL Ag and Urgotul Silver dressing on healing of chronic venous leg ulcers. *Int Wound J.* 2011;9(3):285-94.

67.   Michaels JA, Campbell WB, King BM, Palfreyman SJ, Shackley P, Stevenson M. Randomized controlled trial and cost-effectiveness analysis of silver-donating antimicrobial dressings for venous leg ulcers (VULCAN trial). *Br J Surg.* 2009a;96:1147-56.

68.   Michaels JA, Campbell WB, King BM, et al. A prospective randomised controlled trial and economic modelling of antimicrobial silver dressings versus non-adherent control dressings for venous leg ulcers: the VULCAN trial. *Health Technol Assess.* 2009b;13(56):1-114.

69.   Schuler JJ, Maibenco T, Megerman J, Ware M, Montalvo J. Treatment of chronic venous ulcers using sequential gradient intermittent pneumatic compression. *Phlebology.* 1996;11:111-6.

70.   Ieran M, Zaffuto S, Bagnacani M, Annovi M, Moratti A, Cadossi R. Effect of low frequency pulsing electromagnetic fields on skin ulcers of venous origin in humans: a double-blind study. *J Orthop Res.* 1990;8(2):276-82.

71.   Kenkre JE, Hobbs FD, Carter YH, Holder RL, Holmes EP. A randomized controlled trial of electromagnetic therapy in the primary care management of venous leg ulceration. *Fam Pract.* 1996;13(3):236-41.

72.   Hammarlund C, Sundberg T. Hyperbaric oxygen reduced size of chronic leg ulcers: a randomized double-blind study. *Plast Reconstr Surg.* 1994;93(4):829-33.

73.   Chang DW, Sanchez LA, Veith FJ, Wain RA, Okhi T, Suggs WD. Can a tissue-engineered skin graft improve healing of lower extremity foot wounds after revascularization? *Ann Vasc Surg.* 2000;14(1):44-9.

74.   Brigido SA. The use of an acellular dermal regenerative tissue matrix in the treatment of lower extremity wounds: a prospective 16-week pilot study. *Int Wound J.* 2006;3(3):181-7.

75.   Romanelli M, Dini V, Bertone M, Barbanera S, Brilli C. OASIS wound matrix versus Hyaloskin in the treatment of difficult-to-heal wounds of mixed arterial/venous aetiology. *Int Wound J.* 2007;4(1):3-7.

76.   Romanelli M, Dini V, Bertone MS. Randomized comparison of OASIS wound matrix versus moist wound dressing in the treatment of difficult-to-heal wounds of mixed arterial/venous etiology. *Adv Skin Wound Care.* 2010;23(1):34-8.

77.   Jorgensen B, Price P, Andersen KE, et al. The silver-releasing foam dressing, Contreet Foam, promotes faster healing of critically colonised venous leg ulcers: a randomised, controlled trial. *Int Wound J.* 2005;2(1):64-73.

78.   Miller CN, Newall N, Kapp SE, et al. A randomized-controlled trial comparing cadexomer iodine and nanocrystalline silver on the healing of leg ulcers. *Wound Rep Reg.* 2010;18(4):359-67.

79.   Fumal I, Braham C, Paquet P, Pierard-Franchimont C, Pierard GE. The beneficial toxicity paradox of antimicrobials in leg ulcer healing impaired by a polymicrobial flora: a proof-of-concept study. *Dermatology.* 2002;204 Suppl 1:70-4.

80.   Vuerstaek JD, Vainas T, Wuite J, Nelemans P, Neumann MH, Veraart JC. State-of-the-art treatment of chronic leg ulcers: A randomized controlled trial comparing vacuum-assisted closure (V.A.C.) with modern wound dressings. *J Vasc Surg.* 2006;44(5):1029-37.

81.   Armstrong DG, Lavery LA, Diabetic Foot Study C. Negative pressure wound therapy after partial diabetic foot amputation: a multicentre, randomised controlled trial. *Lancet.* 2005;12;366(9498):1704-10.

82.   Apelqvist J, Armstrong DG, Lavery LA, Boulton AJM. Resource utilization and economic costs of care based on a randomized trial of vacuum-assisted closure therapy in the treatment of diabetic foot wounds. *Am J Surg.* 2008;195:782-8.

83.   Fife CE. Wound Care in the 21st Century. *US Surgery.* 2007:63-64.

84.   Wu SC, Marston W, Armstrong DG. Wound care: the role of advanced wound-healing technologies. *J Am Podiatr Med Assoc.* 2010;100(5):385-94.

85.   Sullivan N, Snyder DL, Tipton K, Uhl S, Schoelles KM. Negative pressure wound therapy devices. *Technology Assessment Report.* Prepared under contract to the Agency for Healthcare Research and Quality (AHRQ), Rockville, MD (Contract No. 290-2007-10063), 2009.

86.   Ubbink DT, Westerbos SJ, Evans D, Land L, Vermeulen H. Topical negative pressure for treating chronic wounds. *Cochrane Database of Systematic Reviews* 2008.Issue 3. Art. No.: CD001989.

87.   Noble-Bell G, Forbes A. A systematic review of the effectiveness of negative pressure wound therapy in the management of diabetes foot ulcers. *Int Wound J.* 2008;5:233-42.

88.   Armstrong DG, Nguyen HC, Lavery LA, van Schie CH, Boulton AJ, Harkless LB. Off-loading the diabetic foot wound: a randomized clinical trial. *Diabetes Care.* 2001;24(6):1019-22.

89.   Katz IA, Harlan A, Miranda-Palma B, et al. A randomized trial of two irremovable off-loading devices in the management of plantar neuropathic diabetic foot ulcers. *Diabetes Care.* 2005;28(3):591-600.

90.   Mustoe TA, O'Shaughnessy K, Kloeters O. Chronic wound pathogenesis and current treatment strategies: a unifying hypothesis. *Plast Reconstr Surg.* 2006;117 Suppl 7:35S-41S.

91. O'Meara S, Cullum NA, Nelson EA. Compression for venous leg ulcers. *Cochrane Database of Systematic Reviews*. 2009 (1):CD000265.

92. Gottrup F, Apelqvist J, Price P. Outcomes in controlled and comparative studies on non-healing wounds: recommendations to improve the quality of evidence in wound management. *J Wound Care*. 2010;19:239-68.

APPENDIX A. THERAPY DESCRIPTIONS AND REFERENCES

Collagen

The term collagen is applied to a species of chemically distinct macromolecular proteins. The variety of collagen structures is one reason for their diverse roles in ulcer healing. The roles of collagen wound products in ulcer healing may be 1) to act as a substrate for hemostasis, 2) chemotaxis to cellular elements of healing such as granulocytes, macrophages, and fibroblasts, 3) to provide a scaffold for more rapid transition to mature collagen production and alignment, or 4) to provide a template for cellular attachment, migration, and proliferation (Purna 2000). FIBRACOL Collagen-Alginate wound dressing (Johnson and Johnson, New Brunswick, NJ) is an advanced wound care device composed of collagen and calcium alginate fibers. It received FDA approval in August of 1998 for topical use for burns and pressure, venous, and diabetic ulcers. Promogran (Johnson and Johnson) consists of 55% collagen and 45% oxidized generated cellulose. It was approved by the FDA in February of 2002. Promogran is an absorbent open-pored, sterile, freeze-dried matrix used as a topical treatment for chronic ulcers including diabetic and venous ulcers. Promogran is composed of natural materials which physically bind to and inactivate damaging proteases while binding and protecting growth factors. (Cullen 2002).

Biological Dressings

This category of wound healing therapies consists of biomaterials made from various components of the extracellular matrix (ECM). These acellular matrices are usually derived from animal or cadaver sources and have undergone processing to remove and retain specific elements of the tissue. A commonly used biologically active dressing, the OASIS Wound Matrix (Cook Biotech, West Lafayette, IN), is an ECM product derived from the small intestinal submucosa of pigs. It received FDA 510(k) approval in 2000 and is indicated for the treatment of diabetic ulcers, venous ulcers, and chronic vascular ulcers, in addition to several other dermatologic conditions. This product retains additional active components found within the ECM, including many growth factors (Hodde 2001; Hodde, 2005; McDevitt, 2003) and several elements of ground substance (Hodde, 1996; McPherson, 1998). OASIS becomes incorporated into the ulcer base and is thought to stimulate ulcer healing by providing a structural scaffold and the growth signals important to complex cellular interactions within ulcers, both of which are dysfunctional and contribute to the persistence of chronic ulcers (Hodde, 2007). Lacking a cellular component, these products have the benefit of a long shelf life and are relatively uncomplicated to administer.

Biological Skin Equivalents (BSE)

These wound-healing therapies are laboratory-derived tissue constructs, designed to resemble various layers of real human skin. They consist of cultured, metabolically active skin cells grown over a scaffold or mesh framework. Two commercially available skin equivalents with FDA approval for treating chronic leg ulcers are Dermagraft and Apligraf. Dermagraft (Advanced BioHealing, Inc., La Jolla, CA) is a dermal tissue substitute that received FDA approval in 2001 for treating diabetic foot ulcers lasting more than 6 weeks. It is formed by culturing human fibroblasts from neonatal foreskin and then growing these fibroblasts over a bioabsorbable polyglactin scaffold. As the cells proliferate *in vitro*, they secrete important components of the extracellular matrix and a large variety of local growth factors (Naughton, 1997). The product is cryopreserved for storage and delivery, but metabolic activity is regained upon thawing and application to the wound bed (Mansbridge, 1998). Apligraf (Organogenesis, Inc., Canton, MA) is a similar skin substitute made from cultured skin cells but is a bilayer construct that contains both dermal and epidermal components. Apligraf (formerly known as Graftskin, Human Skin Equivalent, and Living Skin Equivalent) received FDA approval in 1998 for chronic venous ulcers and in 2000 was granted further approval for use in diabetic foot ulcers. The human cells in both layers, fibroblasts in the dermis and keratinocytes in the epidermis, are derived from purified cultures of neonatal foreskin. The final metabolically active product has a limited shelf life since it is not cryopreserved but delivered "fresh" to sites for clinical use. Both Apligraf and Dermagraft are metabolically active products thought to increase healing by stimulating fibrovascular ingrowth and epithelialization of host tissues (Ehrenreich, 2006; Límová, 2010). They do not "take" like traditional skin grafts that are meant to replace lost tissue with fully functioning skin, but instead become incorporated into the wound bed and stimulate regrowth of the host's own skin tissue (Ehrenreich, 2006; Límová, 2010; Mansbridge, 1999; Phillips, 2002).

Keratinocytes

Keratinocyte-based therapies for wound healing exist in a variety of forms. Use of cultured epidermal keratinocytes to treat chronic leg ulcers was first attempted with autologous (Hefton, 1986; Leigh, 1986) and allogeneic (Leigh, 1987) cells in 1986 and 1987, respectively. Since then, different keratinocyte sources have been utilized; the patient's own skin cells, donor cells from cadavers or patients undergoing cosmetic procedures, and bioengineered "immortalized" keratinocytes have all been used. In addition to using different cellular sources, therapies may vary in their use of fresh, cryopreserved, or lyophilized keratinocytes. These products differ in level of metabolic activity and ease of storage and transportation. Furthermore, various application strategies have been attempted for delivering keratinocytes onto wounds, including various suspension mediums (e.g., fibrin sealant), aerosolized sprays, cellular microcarriers, and gels. These products do not act as grafts or serve as permanent skin replacements, as they are rapidly replaced by the host's own keratinocytes (Kaawach, 1991; Burt, 1989; Auböck, 1988). They are thought to work by stimulating proliferation and migration of host epithelium from wound edges through the production of growth factors and other cytokines (DeLuca, 1992; Duinslaeger, 1994; McKay, 1991). Although there have been multiple studies focusing on keratinocyte use in chronic ulcers, currently the only commercially available products in the U.S. are not indicated for use in leg ulcers. However, there are various products on the market, and with ongoing efforts to expand indications and the continuing research focus in this area, an understanding of the current literature on the topic is important in recognizing the limitations and future expectations of keratinocyte-based wound healing

Platelet-derived Wound Healing - Platelet-derived Growth Factors (PDGF)

Human platelet-derived growth factor is a substance naturally produced by the body to help in wound healing. It works by helping to repair and replace dead skin and other tissues, attracting cells that repair wounds, and helping to close and heal the ulcers. (Pierce 1991). Regranex Gel (becaplermin 0.01%, Johnson & Johnson, New Brunswick, NJ) was approved by the FDA in 1997 for the treatment of diabetic foot ulcers. Regranex is a genetically engineered product that mimics PDGF in the body. It is indicated for treating lower-extremity neuropathic ulcers that extend into the subcutaneous tissue or beyond, but which have an adequate blood supply. It is intended for use as an adjunct to traditional ulcer care strategies, such as initial sharp debridement, daily dressing changes, pressure relief and treatment of infection if present (Label indication 1997).

Platelet Rich Plasma

Platelet-rich plasma (PRP) is derived from newly drawn whole blood prepared by specialized centrifugation to create plasma having a platelet concentration above baseline. PRPs themselves are have been used in wound healing since 1985 and do not require FDA approval, but centrifuges used to spin whole blood for the creation of PRP do require approval. PRP contains a high level of platelets and a full complement of clotting and growth factors which aid in healing by attracting undifferentiated cells and activating cell division (Lacci 2010). Autologel System (Cytomedix Inc) received FDA approval in September of 2007 and consists of a table top centrifuge (AutoloGel II Centrifuge) and blood access and processing devices.

Silver

The therapeutic potential of silver has long been recognized, and reports of its use in chronic ulcers have been documented in surgical textbooks as early as 1617 (Klasen, 2000). Due to the broad bactericidal action of silver (Ip, 2006) and the understanding that wound healing is impaired when bacterial levels surpass a particular threshold (Bowler, 2001), multiple silver-based products have been developed to aid in wound healing. These products incorporate silver into topical creams (silver sulfadiazine or Silvadene; King Pharmaceuticals, Bristol, TN) or within various types of dressings, including foams (Contreet Ag; Coloplast, Marietta, GA), hydrocolloids (Contreet H; Coloplast, Marietta, GA), hydrofibers (Aquacel-Ag; Covatec, Skillman, NJ), alginates (Silvercel; Systagenix, Quincy, MA), film polymers (Arglaes; Medline, Mundelein, IL), and a polyethylene mesh with nanocrystalline silver (Acticoat-7; Smith and Nephew, Hull, UK). These products work through the release of reactive silver cations, [Ag^+], which may disrupt components of the bacterial cell wall, inhibit microbial respiratory enzymes and elements of the electron transport chain, and impair the synthesis and function of DNA and RNA (Atiyeh, 2007). Although these effects are desirable when directed against bacterial and fungal organisms, it is important to recognize the indiscriminant action of silver. Cytotoxicity of various host cells, including keratinocytes and fibroblasts, has been shown to occur from silver, and a delicate balance exists between the beneficial decrease in bacterial burden and the deleterious effects on host cells that can also delay wound closure (Atiyeh, 2007; Poon, 2004; Hollinger, 1996)

Intermittent Pneumatic Compression Therapy

Intermittent pneumatic compression (IPC) therapy is delivered through inflatable, single-patient-use, garments containing one or more air chambers. Garments are applied to the foot, calf, or calf and thigh and intermittently inflated and deflated with air by means of a powered pneumatic pump to simulate the normal ambulatory calf and foot pump. This action propels the blood of the deep veins towards the heart and benefits the non-ambulatory patient by increasing blood flow velocity in the deep veins and reducing stasis, decreasing venous hypertension, flushing valve pockets, and decreasing interstitial edema (Comerota 2011). Pneumatic compression devices are cleared for marketing under the FDA 510(k) process as Class II devices intended for use in prevention of blood pooling in a limb by periodically inflating a sleeve around the limb. No clinical data was needed for FDA approval since they existed prior to the passage of the Medical Device Amendments of 1976.

Negative Pressure Wound Therapy (NPWT)

NPWT, also referred to as "vacuum assisted wound closure," is the process of creating a tightly sealed dressing around a wound and using a suction pump to apply a sub-atmospheric (or "negative") pressure evenly across the surface in a continuous or intermittent manner (Venturi, 2005). A drainage canister is attached to store fluid collected from wound suction. The first FDA approved, commercially available NPWT product was the Vacuum Assisted Closure™ device (Kinetic Concepts, Inc., San Antonio, TX), introduced to the market in 1995. Since then, the approved indications for its use have continually expanded and currently include diabetic foot ulcers, venous leg ulcers, and pressure ulcers, as well as several non-ulcerative conditions. Other NPWT devices include the Versatile 1™ (BlueSky Medical, Carlsbad, CA), which received FDA approval in 2004, and the Renasys™EZ and Renasys™Go (Smith and Nephew Inc., Largo, FL), approved in 2008 and 2009, respectively. These devices are proposed to enhance wound healing by increasing granulation tissue and local perfusion (Morykwas, 1997), reducing tissue edema, decreasing bacterial load (Morykwas, 1997), and stimulating cellular proliferation via induction of mechanical stress (Olenius, 1993; Saxena, 2004). NPWT may be used as either a primary treatment to achieve complete wound healing, or as a temporary therapy to prepare a wound so that another treatment can be attempted to achieve complete wound closure.

Electromagnetic Therapy (EMT)

EMT utilizes the electrical field created between large, oppositely charged capacitors or, more commonly, the electrical field that develops from exposure to an oscillating magnetic field (Lee, 1993). There are various potential mechanisms by which EMT may enhance wound healing. Normal human skin has been found to produce a steady state transcutaneous electrical potential (Foulds, 1983) that, upon epithelial disruption, short-circuits to produce an endogenous electrical current (Burr, 1940; Illingworth, 1980; Nuccitelli, 2003; Zhao, 2006) and a resultant electrical field (Nuccitelli, 2003; Zhao, 2006). This wound-induced electrical field has been shown to regulate cell division in wound healing (Song, 2002) and to guide the cellular migration through specific signaling pathways (Zhao, 2006; Fang, 1999). EMT is thought to work by mimicking or enhancing these natural wound-induced electrical fields. No EMT devices have received FDA approval for use in chronic wounds; however, these products have received approval for other indications and are commercially available. Despite the lack of FDA approval, the Centers for Medicare and Medicaid Services (CMS) has deemed EMT to be a reasonable adjuvant treatment for chronic ulcers of diabetic, venous, and arterial etiologies. Because of this, CMS covers the use of EMT for chronic ulcers not responding to standard care.

Hyperbaric Oxygen Therapy (HBOT)

HBOT involves the use of specialized compression chambers capable of delivering increased concentrations of oxygen (usually 100% O_2) under elevated atmospheric pressures (usually 1.5-3.0 ATA). This greatly increases systemic levels of oxygen (Sheffield, 1985), achieving arterial oxygen tensions upwards of 2000 mmHg (normally 100 mmHg) and tissue oxygen tensions up to 500 mmHg (normally 55 mmHg) (Gill, 2004). Individual treatment sessions usually last between 45 and 120 minutes and may be done once or twice a day for a total of 10-30 sessions. HBOT is FDA approved for a dynamic list of indications, including wound healing, as deemed appropriate by the Undersea and Hyperbaric Medical Society. Examples of devices include the OxyHeal 1000 Monoplace Hyperbaric Chamber (OxyHeal Health Group, LaJolla, CA) and the Multiplace Hyperbaric Chambers (Makai Marine Industries, Inc., Boca Raton, FL), which received FDA approval in 2005 and 2004 respectively. The role oxygen plays in the process of normal wound healing is complex. Although hypoxia stimulates certain steps in wound healing (Knighton, 1983; Jensen, 1986), and the low oxygen levels in the center of a wound are important in initiating repair (Thackham, 2008), many key aspects of wound healing are oxygen dependent (Gordillo, 2003). These include collagen deposition (Jonsson, 1991), angiogenesis (Hopf, 2005), fibroblast and endothelial cell proliferation (Tompach, 1997), and bacterial clearance (Knighton, 1986; Allen, 1997; Hopf, 1997; Greif, 2000). By raising arterial oxygen tension and the blood-oxygen level delivered to a chronic wound (Rollins, 2006), HBOT is thought not only to supply a missing nutrient but also to promote the oxygen dependent steps in wound healing, to up regulate local growth factors (Thom, 2009), and to down regulate inhibitory cytokines (Thom, 2009). Although thought to be a relatively safe treatment, this delivery of concentrated oxygen in a compression chamber can be complicated by the increased pressure (e.g. ear and sinus barotrauma) or oxygen toxicity (e.g. acute cerebral toxicity and chronic pulmonary toxicity) (Plafki 2000; Sheffield, 2003).

Topical Oxygen Therapy (TOT)

Similar to HBOT, this category of products aims to promote ulcer healing by correcting the low oxygen levels found within chronic wounds. TOT was developed in an effort to overcome drawbacks inherent with HBOT and works to promote wound oxygenation through a physiological distinct mechanism. While HBOT uses a compression chamber to systemically deliver high O_2 levels under an elevated atmospheric pressure, TOT works by covering a wound with an airtight bag or chamber and using a portable device to fill the container with concentrated oxygen. Although this results in very slight elevations in local pressure (usually 1.004 - 1.013 ATA), this is far less than the levels reached in HBOT (up to 2.5 - 3.0 ATA) and is not considered truly "hyperbaric" (Feldmeier, 2005). TOT is thought to increase local oxygen levels by simple diffusion of the externally applied gas into superficial wound tissues (Fries, 2005). This method of wound oxygenation may induce angiogenesis through upregulation of specific growth factors (Gordillo, 2008; Scott, 2005) and has been postulated to promote cell motility, extracellular matrix formation, and angiogenesis by correcting hypoxia at the wound center (Gordillo, 2003). Examples of these products include the Hyper-Box Topical Wound Oxygen System (Qualtech House, Gateway, Ireland) that received FDA approval in 2008 and EpiFlo (Ogenix, Corp., Beachwood, OH), most recently approved in 2012 for chronic skin ulcerations due to diabetes and venous stasis. Although CMS covers use of HBOT in some chronic wounds, it does not reimburse for TOT.

Ozone Oxygen Therapy

Ozone is an oxidizing agent. When ozone molecules are administered via gas or liquid, the ozone is theorized to promote tissue healing. Healthy cells are reported to survive and multiply while defective cells, bacteria, and viruses are destroyed. Ozone has been used to treat medical conditions since the late 19th century, however, there is little known about its safety and efficacy. Ozone can be administered to chronic wounds using a technique known as ozone bagging, a technique in which the effected limb is sealed for up to two hours in a bag containing ozone. Alternatively, ozone-enriched water or vegetable oil may be applied to the skin. Opinions are mixed about the safety of ozone therapy. While some advocates suggest that there is a very low risk of side effects the fact that it is a toxic gas has caused others to question the safety. (Intelihealth, Natural Standard)

References

Allen DB, Maguire JJ, Mahdavian M, et al. Wound hypoxia and acidosis limit neutrophil bacterial killing mechanisms. *Arch Surg.* 1997;132:991-6.

Atiyeh BS, Costagliola M, Hayek SN, Dibo SA. Effect of silver on burn wound infection control and healing: Review of the literature. *Burns.* 2007;33(2):139-48.

Auböck J, Irschick E, Romani N, et al. Rejection, after a slightly prolonged survival time, of Langerhans cell-free allogeneic cultured epidermis used for wound coverage in humans. *Transplantation.* 1988;45:730-7.

Bowler PG, Duerdon B, Armstrong DG. Wound microbiology and associated approaches to wound Management. *Clin Microbiol Rev.* 2001;14:244-69.

Burr HS, Taffel M, Harvey SC. An electrometric study of the healing wound in man. *Yale J Biol Med.* 1940;12:483-5.

Burt AM, Pallet CD, Sloane JP, et al. Survival of cultured allografts in patients with burns assessed with a probe specific for Y chromosome. *BMJ.* 1989;298:915-7.

Comerota AJ. Intermittent pneumatic compression: physiologic and clinical basis to improve management of venous leg ulcers. *J Vasc Surg.* 2011;53(4):1121-9.

Cullen B, Smith R, McCulloch E, Silcock D, Morrison L. Mechanism of action of Promogran, a protease modulating matrix, for treatment of diabetic foot ulcers. *Wound Repair Regen.* 2002;10(1):16-25.

DeLuca M, Albanese E, Cancedda R, et al. Treatment of leg ulcers with cryopreserved allogeneic cultured epithelium. *Arch Dermatol.* 1992;128:633-8.

Duinslaeger L, Verbeken G, Reper P, Delaey B, Vanhalle S, Vanderkelen A. Lyophilized keratinocyte cell lysates contain multiple mitogenic activities and stimulate closure of meshed skin auto-graft-covered burn wounds with efficiency to that of fresh allogeneic keratinocyte cultures. *Plast Reconstr Surg.* 1994;98:110-7.

Ehrenreich M, Ruszczak Z. Update on tissue-engineered biological dressings. *Tissue Eng.* 2006;12:1-18.

Fang KS, Ionides E, Oster G, Nuccitelli R, Isseroff RR. Epidermal growth factor receptor relocalization and kinase activity are necessary for directional migration of keratinocytes in DC electric fields. *J Cell Sci.* 1999;112(12):1967-78.

Feldmeier JJ, Hopf HW, Warriner RA 3rd, Fife CE, Gesell LB, and Bennett M. UHMS position statement: topical oxygen for chronic wounds. *Undersea Hyperb Med.* 2005;32:157-68.

Foulds IS, Barker AT. Human skin battery potentials and their possible role in wound healing. *Br J Dermatol.* 1983;109:515-22.

Fries RB, Wallace WA, Roy S. Dermal excisional wound healing in pigs following treatment with topically applied pure oxygen. *Mutat Res.* 2005;579:172-81.

Gill AL, Bell CN. Hyperbaric oxygen: its uses, mechanisms of action and outcomes. *Q J Med.* 2004;97:385-95.

Gordillo GM, Roy S, Khanna S, et al. Topical oxygen therapy induces vascular endothelial growth factor expression and improves closure of clinically presented chronic wounds. *Clin Exp Pharmacol Physiol.* 2008;35:957-64.

Gordillo GM, Sen CK. Revisiting the essential role of oxygen in wound healing. *Am J Surg.* 2003;186:259-63.

Greif R, Akca O, Horn E-P, Kurz A, Sessler D I. Supplemental perioperative oxygen to reduce the incidence of surgical-wound infection. *N Engl J Med.* 2000;342:161–7.

Hefton JM, Caldwell D, Biozes DG et al. Grafting of skin ulcers with cultured autologous epidermal cells. *J Am Acad Dermatol.* 1986;14:399-405.

Hodde JP, Badylak SF, Brightman AO, Voytik-Harbin SL. Glycosaminoglycan content of small intestinal submucosa: a bioscaffold for tissue replacement. *Tissue Eng.* 1996;2:209-17.

Hodde JP, Ernst DM, Hiles MC. An investigation of the long-term bioactivity of endogenous growth factor in OASIS Wound Matrix. *J Wound Care.* 2005;14(1):23-5.

Hodde JP, Hiles MC. Bioactive FGF-2 in sterilized extracellular matrix. *Wounds.* 2001;13:195-201.

Hodde JP, Johnson CE. Extracellular matrix as a strategy for treating chronic wounds. *Am J Clin Dermatol.* 2007;8(2):61-6.

Hollinger, MA. Toxicological aspects of topical silver pharmaceuticals. *Crit Rev Toxicol.* 1996;26:255-60.

Hopf HW, Gibson JJ, Angeles AP, et al. Hyperoxia and angiogenesis. *Wound Rep Reg.* 2005;13:558-64.

Hopf HW, Hunt TK, West JM, et al. Wound tissue oxygen tension predicts the risk of wound infection in surgical patients. *Arch Surg.* 1997;132:997-1005.

Illingworth CM, Barker AT. Measurement of electrical currents emerging during the regeneration of amputated fingertips in children. *Clin Phys Physiol Meas.* 1980;1:87-9.

Intelihealth.com. Ozone therapy. Available at: http://www.intelihealth.com/IH/ihtIH/ WSIHW000/8513/34968/358849.html?d=dmtContent. Accessed October 1, 2012.

Ip M, Lui SL, Poon VKM, Lung I, Burd A. Antimicrobial activities of silver dressings: an in vitro comparison. *J Med Microbiol.* 2006;55:59-63.

Jensen JA, Hunt TK, Scheuenstuhl H, Banda MJ. Effect of lactate, pyruvate and pH on secretion of angiogenesis and mitogenesis factors by macrophages. *Lab Invest.* 1986;54:574-8.

Jonsson K, Jensen JA, Goodson WH III, et al. Tissue oxygenation, anemia, and perfusion in relation to wound healing in surgical patients. *Ann Surg.* 1991;214:605-13.

Kaawach WF, Oliver AM, Weiler-Mithoff E, Abramovich DR, Rayner CR. Survival assessment of cultured epidermal allografts applied onto partial-thickness burn wounds. *Br J Plast Surg.* 1991;44:321-4.

Klasen HJ. Historical review of the use of silver in the treatment of burns. I. Early uses. *Burns.* 2000;26:117-30.

Knighton DR, Halliday B, Hunt TK. Oxygen as an antibiotic. A comparison of the effects of inspired oxygen concentration and antibiotic administration on in vivo bacterial clearance. *Arch Surg.* 1986;121:191-5.

Knighton DR, Hunt TK, Scheuenstuhl H, Halliday BJ, Werb Z, Banda MJ. Oxygen tension regulates the expression of angiogenesis factor by macrophages. *Science.* 1983;221:1283-5.

Lacci KM, Dardik A. Platelet-rich plasma: support for its use in wound healing. *Yale J Biol Med.* 2010.83(1):1-9

Lee RC, Canaday DJ, Doong H. A review of the biophysical basis for the clinical application of electric fields in soft-tissue repair. *J Burn Care Rehabil.* 1993;14:319-35.

Leigh IM, Purkis PE. Culture grafted leg ulcers. *Clin Exp Dermatol.* 1986;11:650-2.

Leigh IM, Purkis PE, Navsaria HA, Phillips TJ. Treatment of chronic venous leg ulcers with sheets of cultured allogenic keratinocytes. *Br J Dermatol.* 1987;117:591-7.

Límová M. Active wound coverings: bioengineered skin and dermal substitutes. *Surg Clin North Am.* 2010;90(6):1237-55.

Mansbridge J, Liu K, Patch R, et al. Three-dimensional fibroblast culture implant for the treatment of diabetic foot ulcers: metabolic activity and therapeutic range. *Tissue Eng.* 1998;4:403-14.

Mansbridge JN, Liu K, Pinney RE, Patch R, Ratcliffe A, Naughton GK. Growth factors secreted by fibroblasts: role in healing diabetic foot ulcers. *Diabetes, Obes Metabol.* 1999;1:265-79.

McDevitt CA, Wildey GM, Cutrone RM. Transforming growth factor beta*1* in a sterilized tissue derived from the pig small intestine submucosa. *J Biomed Mater Res.* 2003;67A:637-40.

McKay IA, Leigh IM. Epidermal cytokines and their roles in cutaneous wound healing. *Br J Dermatol.* 1991;124:513-8.

McPherson TB, Badylak SF. Characterization of fibronectin derived from porcine small intestinal submucosa. *Tissue Eng.* 1998;4:75-83.

Morykwas MJ, Argenta LC, Shelton-Brown EI, et al. Vacuum-assisted closure: a new method for wound control and treatment: animal studies and basic foundation. *Ann Plast Surg.* 1997;38(6):553-62.

Natural Standard Professional Monograph. Ozone therapy. 2012. Available at: http://www. naturalstandard.com/databases/hw/ozone.asp?. Accessed October 1, 2012.

Naughton G, Mansbridge J, Gentzkow G. A metabolically active human dermal replacement for the treatment of diabetic foot ulcers. *Artificial Organs.* 1997;21:1203-10.

Nuccitelli R. A role for endogenous electric fields in wound healing. *Curr Top Dev Biol.* 2003;58:1-26.

Olenius M, Dalsgaard C, Wickman M. Mitotic activity in the expanded human skin. *Plast Reconstr Surg.* 1993;91:213-6.

Phillips TJ, Manzoor J, Rojas A, et al. The longevity of a bilayered skin substitute after application to venous ulcers. *Arch Dermatol*. 2002;138:1079-81.

Pierce GF et al. Role of platelet-derived growth factor in wound healing. *J Cell Biochem*. 1991;45 (4):319-26.

Plafki C, Peters P, Almeling M, Welslau W, Busch R. Complications and side effects of hyperbaric oxygen therapy. *Aviat Space Environ Med*. 2000;71:119-24.

Poon VK, Burd A. In vitro cytotoxity of silver: implication for clinical wound care. *Burns*. 2004;30:140-7.

Purna S., Babu M. Collagen based dressings – A review. *Burns*, 2000:26:54-62.

Regranex Product Label. www.accessdata.fda.gov/drugsatfda_docs/label/1997/becaomj121697-lab.pdf. Accessed June 15, 2012.

Rollins MD, Gibson JJ, Hunt TK, Hopf HW. Wound oxygen levels during hyperbaric oxygen treatment in healing wounds. *Undersea Hyperb Med*. 2006;33:17-25.

Saxena V, Hwang CW, Huang S, et al. Vacuum-assisted closure: microdeformations of wounds and cell proliferation. *Plast Reconstr Surg*. 2004;114(5):1086-96.

Scott GF, Reeves RE. Topical Oxygen Alters Angiogenesis-Related Growth Factor Expression in Chronic Diabetic Foot Ulcers. *Wound Repair Regen*. 2005;13:A4-A27.

Sheffield PJ. Tissue oxygen measurements with respect to soft-tissue wound healing with normobaric and hyperbaric oxygen. *HBO Rev*. 1985;6:18-46.

Sheffield PJ, Sheffield JC. Complication rates for hyperbaric oxygen therapy patients and their attendants: a 22 year analysis. In: Proceedings of the Fourteenth International Congress on Hyperbaric Medicine. 2003:312-8.

Song B, Zhao M, Forrester JV, McCaig CD. Electrical cues regulate the orientation and frequency of cell division and the rate of wound healing in vivo. *Proc Natl Acad. Sci USA*. 2002;99:13577-82.

Thackham JA, McElwain DLS, Long RJ. The use of hyperbaric oxygen therapy to treat chronic wounds: a review. *Wound Repair Regen*. 2008;16:321-30.

Thom SR. Oxidative stress is fundamental to hyperbaric oxygen therapy. *J Appl Physiol*. 2009;106:988-95.

Tompach PC, Lew D, Stoll JL. Cell response to hyperbaric oxygen treatment. *Int J Oral Maxillofac Surg*. 1997;26:82-6.

Venturi ML, Attinger CE, Mesbahi AN, Hess CL, Graw KS. Mechanisms and clinical applications of the vacuum-assisted closure (VAC) device: a review. *Am J Clin Dermatol*. 2005;6:185-94.

Zhao, M. *et al*. Electrical signals control wound healing through phosphatidylinositol-3-OH kinase-γ and PTEN. *Nature*. 2006;442:457-60.

APPENDIX B. SEARCH STRATEGY

Search Strategy:

1	exp Skin Ulcer/ (31597)
2	exp Foot Ulcer/ (5874)
3	exp Leg Ulcer/ (15666)
4	exp Varicose Ulcer/ (3490)
5	exp Diabetic Foot/ (4864)
6	exp Wound Healing/ (83186)
7	exp Venous Insufficiency/ (5352)
8	or/1-7 (114315)

9   limit 8 to (clinical trial, all or clinical trial, phase i or clinical trial, phase ii or clinical trial, phase iii or clinical trial, phase iv or clinical trial or controlled clinical trial or meta analysis or randomized controlled trial) (6955)

10	randomized controlled trial.pt. (321315)
11	controlled clinical trial.pt. (83663)
12	random*.ti,ab. (545362)
13	placebo.ti,ab. (132724)
14	or/10-13 (736326)
15	(animals not (humans and animals)).sh. (3590935)
16	14 not 15 (659693)
17	8 and 16 (5990)

18   9 or 17 (8200)

19   limit 18 to (english language and humans and yr="1995 -Current") (5646) [a few more important limits]

20	artificial skin.mp. or exp Skin, Artificial/ (1844)
21	19 and 20 (65)
22	biological dressings.mp. or exp Biological Dressings/ (1128)
23	19 and 22 (38)
24	exp Negative-Pressure Wound Therapy/ or exp Lower Body Negative Pressure/ or negative pressure.mp. (5422)
25	19 and 24 (84)
26	exp Collagen/ or collagen.mp. (145508)
27	19 and 26 (287)
28	exp Silver/ or exp Silver Proteins/ or silver.mp. (37481)
29	19 and 28 (105)
30	exp Oxygen/ or topical oxygen.mp. (134274)
31	19 and 30 (51)
32	exp Hyperbaric Oxygenation/ or hyperbaric oxygen*.mp. (10425)
33	19 and 32 (62)
34	electromagnet*.mp. or exp Electromagnetic Phenomena/ (311999)

35   19 and 34 (55)
36   exp Platelet-Derived Growth Factor/ or platelet-derived.mp. or exp Growth Substances/ (570646)
37   19 and 36 (179)
38   exp Platelet-Rich Plasma/ or platelet-rich.mp. (5704)
39   19 and 38 (66)
40   exp Intermittent Pneumatic Compression Devices/ or pneumatic compress*.mp. or compress* therapy.mp. or compress* pump.mp. (1625)
41   19 and 40 (130)
42   21 or 23 or 25 or 27 or 29 or 31 or 33 or 35 or 37 or 39 or 41 (1014)

APPENDIX C. PEER REVIEW COMMENTS/AUTHOR RESPONSES

REVIEWER COMMENT	RESPONSE
1. Are the objectives, scope, and methods for this review clearly described?	
Yes	
Yes	
Yes	
Yes	
Yes	
Yes. This report represents a monumental work effort. It is, in my judgment, the most comprehensive and objective review I have seen to date. The persons who prepared this report are to be commended for their efforts.	Thank you.
2. Is there any indication of bias in our synthesis of the evidence?	
Not sure that like was compared to like. I would worry about your RCT grading system if RCTs used for FDA approval (PDGF and synthetic skin) are graded lower than a NPWT study that was not really blinded. I also worry at all of your studies did not treat similar groups of individuals. For example, the HBO RCTs were very inconsistent with respect to the Wagner grade.	We assigned grades based on established criteria for evaluating risk of bias in RCTs. These criteria may be different than criteria for FDA approval.

We agree that the populations varied from study to study and attempted to clarify that in the description of the studies. |
No	
No	
No (reviewer provided citation for Lancet article [2012] on spray-applied cell therapy)	Thank you. We reviewed this citation. The treatment is not FDA approved (this was a phase 2 trial) and therefore is not eligible for inclusion in our review.
No	
No	
3. Are there any published or unpublished studies that we may have overlooked?	
Yes – total contact cast literature	We did not consider total contact casting to be an "advanced wound care product." Although it may be an important therapeutic option, it was not recommended by our topic stakeholders and is outside the scope of our review.
No	
No	

REVIEWER COMMENT	RESPONSE
Yes Considering collagen dressings as a stand-alone category presents challenges as they are frequently used as deliver vehicles for silver, growth factors, protease inhibitors, etc. This should be acknowledged as a limitation. As such there may be other studies to be considered for inclusion under collagen [1-5]; apligraf [6]; and silver.[2] 1. Blume, P., et al., Formulated collagen gel accelerates healing rate immediately after application in patients with diabetic neuropathic foot ulcers. Wound Repair & Regeneration, 2011. 19(3): p. 302-8. 2. Gottrup, F., et al., Collagen/ORC/silver treatment of diabetic foot ulcers; A randomised controlled trial. Wound Repair and Regeneration, 2011. 19(2): p. A24. 3. Letendre, S., et al., Pilot trial of biovance collagen-based wound covering for diabetic ulcers. Advances in Skin & Wound Care, 2009. 22(4): p. 161-6. 4. Motzkau, M., et al., Expression of matrix-metalloproteases in the fluid of chronic diabetic foot wounds treated with a protease absorbent dressing. Experimental & Clinical Endocrinology & Diabetes, 2011. 119(5): p. 286-90. 5. Mulder, G., et al., Treatment of nonhealing diabetic foot ulcers with a platelet-derived growth factor gene-activated matrix (GAM501): results of a phase 1/2 trial. Wound Repair & Regeneration, 2009. 17(6): p. 772-9. 6. Sams, H.H., J. Chen, and L.E. King, Graftskin treatment of difficult to heal diabetic foot ulcers: one center's experience. Dermatologic Surgery, 2002. 28(8): p. 698-703	We have clarified that the studies included in the collagen section are studies of an inert collagen matrix product. We have reviewed the suggested references: 1. This trial has been added. 2. An abstract – not eligible for inclusion (we were unable to find the data in a peer-reviewed publication) 3. A case series – not eligible for inclusion 4. This study has been mentioned in the collagen section but due to a difference in the goal of the study and incomplete reporting is not given as much attention as other trials 5. A "cohort" study – not eligible for inclusion 6. This report presents data from one site of a multisite trial that is included in the report (Veves 2001)
No. To the best of my knowledge, this report appears to have reviewed all of the pertinent information relevant to the topics studied.	Thank you
4. Please write any additional suggestions or comments below. If applicable, please indicate the page and line numbers from the draft report.	
I am concerned that the device assessments were not as rigorous as the FDA approved products. Care needs to be made in recommendations. Also you did assess that HBO was inferior to shockwave and therapy that was later shown in the US to not be superior to standard off-loading of diabetic feet.	We identified and discussed one HBO trial conducted in Taiwan that directly compared HBO to shockwave therapy. We did not identify any trials meeting our inclusion criteria that directly compared shockwave therapy to standard off-loading of diabetic feet. We have added a paragraph with results from strictly controlled off-loading studies for comparison purposes.
Please see my comments within the body of the paper. (*Investigator NOTE: comments from body of paper have been added to list below*) The first 18 pages of the document need major revisions. After page 18, the material is written in more scientific manner which it appears more accurate than what is presented on the first initial pages. a. Page 1 Please define what you mean by diabetic ulcers. Arterial and venous ulcers can also happen in diabetic patients. How about neuropathic ulcers? Were they studied or reported in this paper? b. Page 1 Is your paper focused only on foot ulcers? Most venous ulcers occur in the legs. When studying the effectiveness of a device, please be more specific on location of the ulcers where the product was used.	The first 18 pages of the document are the executive summary and we attempted to condense a great deal of information into a more readable format. As the reviewer has noted, there are many important details about the studies and we have attempted to include the essential elements in the executive summary without simply repeating the full text of the report. a. The studies included in the section on diabetic ulcers are studies of populations described by the study authors as having diabetic ulcers. Diabetic ulcers are caused by peripheral neuropathy and/or peripheral vascular disease. The most common cause of neuropathic ulcers is diabetes and many of these studies included only patients with neuropathic ulcers. Most studies excluded patients with inadequate circulation. We have added that information to the report when it was provided by the study authors. b. The paper is not focused on foot ulcers. We have added the location of the ulcers (an overview in the executive summary and more information in the body of the report).

REVIEWER COMMENT	RESPONSE
c. Page 1 How about the impact of PVD and plantar pressures? I can heal a wound that is neuropathic or has infection as long as there is blood flow to the tissue!!!!	c. As noted in the overview of studies for KQ1, only one trial enrolled patients with strictly ischemic diabetic ulcers; in 27 of 35 trials, the ulcers were either neuropathic or patients with vascular disease were excluded.
d. Page 1 I am not sure that the statement "venous disease accounts for the majority of chronic ulcers" is correct. Venous ulcers is seen mostly on non-American populations, but current research shows occurrence of PAD related ulcers in US population	d. This statement is correct. In the US, venous disease is responsible for 72% of leg ulcers, mixed venous and arterial disease for 22%, and pure arterial disease for about 6%. References have been added.
e. Page 1 Please define what you mean by diabetic ulcers? Are these patients who are diabetic with normal arterial, venous and nerve supplies? How are these patient populations different than those who have "arterial" ulcers or "venous ulcers?	e. As noted in item "a" above, we categorized studies based on the study authors' descriptions of their included populations. We have added an overview of the studies which shows that, in most cases, studies of patients with diabetic ulcers excluded patients with inadequate blood flow. We recognize that patients with diabetes who are judged to have "adequate circulation" via clinical examination including pulses and blood pressure assessment may have microvascular arterial insufficiency. Nonetheless, we have categorized patients according to authors' definitions and included descriptions of the individual studies.
f. Page 3. Is this study shared with Dr. Robbins, our VA Central Office Chief of Podiatry? He needs to be informed on this study as this study can impact the podiatry field at the VA tremendously. His input on who should review this paper is important.	f. Dr. Robbins was a member of the Technical Expert Panel for the report, provided input on the key questions, scope of review, study inclusion criteria and outcomes of interest (including categorization of populations and interventions) and has reviewed the report.
g. Page 3 – overview of sizes of ulcers – Where are these ulcers? On the leg/shin area? Dorsal foot? Plantar foot? Each location will respond differently to different wound care product)	g. We have added location to the overview of the studies. We also added this information to the results section in the full report and in the executive summary if there appeared to be differences in outcomes based on ulcer location.
h. Page 3 – KQ1 (diabetic ulcers) – Did all the subject studied for this question have normal blood flow and sensate feet?	h. We have added this information to the overview of the studies.
i. Page 4 – Collagen – Were there any beneficial effect in using collagen? Are you then telling the reader that using collagen on wounds is a waste of money? Is there any wound type that collagen can be helpful, i.e., draining wound? As a reader, I get the conclusion that I will be wasting my money and time if I used collagen. Is that what you want your readers to get out of this paragraph?	i. One study of collagen as a matrix material found a benefit for ulcer healing. We have clarified that other treatments may use collagen as a vehicle for delivery of the active substance (e.g., silver).
j. Page 4 – Biological Dressings – Did all the subjects have normal blood flow? Please define what you mean by biological dressing. Are these different than biological skin equivalents?	j. One study excluded patients with severe arterial disease and the other included only patients with adequate circulation. We have defined biological dressings as acellular matrices with a biologically active component. We have defined biological skin equivalents as tissue constructs designed to resemble layers of human skin.
k. Page 4 – Biological Skin Equivalents – a) I am not sure what you mean metabolically active dermagraft. As a practitioner who uses dermagraft, I have never heard of this terminology. b) It is helpful to include how many (in average) dermagraft or apligraf application took in order to heal the wounds, as there is always the cost of care than can also impact treatment regimen used. Also in the past we were told that one application of apligraf was enough to get the wound to heal but now they are recommending weekly applications. The same goes for dermagraft. When dermagraft first hit the market, we could only use it up to 3 applications and now it is up to 7 applications. It is important to include how many graft applications these studies used in order to get the reported results.	k. The finding about metabolically active dermagraft was from an early trial (Naughton 1997). They found that some samples had lower metabolic activity (non-therapeutic range) and suggest that, as a result, the manufacturing process was modified to ensure that all samples have an appropriate therapeutic level. We have clarified this. We have also added information about the number of applications to the full report
l. Page 5 – Platelet-rich Plasma – Please add how many applications of PRP it took to get the wound to heal? Was it daily, weekly, monthly application?	l. We have added this information to the executive summary and the report.
m. Page 5 – Silver Products – Please be more specific as to exact type of silver products used. The silver ointment used for many years is silvadene cream which is cheaper than most other wound products. Now we have so many silver dressings with nano and micro size silver in it and each product is different based on its technology! So not all silver products are the same. The paragraph above can be very misleading, does not have any scientific value to it as it does not specify which specific silver technology you are referring to.	m. This information is in the main report and has now been clarified in the executive summary.

REVIEWER COMMENT	RESPONSE
n. Page 5 – NPWT – Please be more specific. How much better improvement? 50%? , 60%, 70% better? Was it significantly or marginally better? How about time to gain complete healing? Or was this study based on wound reduction size only.	n. We have added the absolute risk difference for NPWT and the other treatments.
Page 6-7 – KQ1 summary a) under Secondary Outcomes – were these ulcers "diabetic ulcers" or "arterial" ulcers? b) The above summary does not cover the answer to all of the questions specifically "Is efficacy dependent on ancillary therapies?" – not clearly covered for each individual treatment regimen and "Does efficacy differ according to patient demographics, comorbid conditions, treatment compliance, or activity level?" – not clearly covered for each individual treatment regimen	o. We found significant improvement in percentage of ulcers healed with Apligraf for both diabetic and venous ulcers. We did not review FDA reasoning behind their approval process (which may have included studies and data not available or eligible for this report) and make no statement regarding their approval.
o. Page 7 – Biological Skin Equivalents – The comments above contradict the FDA reported studies. Apligraf was initially approved by the FDA in 1998 for use in venous ulcers. Later, its indication expended to include arterial/diabetic ulcers in 2000. So is FDA wrong?	p. We have added this information.
p. Page 8 – Silver Products – please be specific on type of silver dressing used	q. The IPC trial did not report time to healing or ulcer recurrence.
q. Page 8 – Intermittent Pneumatic Compression Therapy – How about time to healing? Did the IPC reduce the time to healing? How about ulcer recurrence rate?	r. We agree that arterial ulcers and treatment for these are important. However, we identified only one trial specifically focused on arterial ulcers. We noted in the text that some of the patients in the diabetic ulcer studies may have had microvascular disease despite the fact that most studies excluded patients with macrovascular disease. Similarly, patients may have had mixed venous and arterial disease. This is an important area requiring future research.
r. Page 10 – KQ3 – How come this is different than the answers to other questions above? Are not there device/product-specific studies for arterial ulcers? How about use of collagen? skin substitutes i.e., apligraf? How about HBO therapy? PRP? This section is too brief and does not do the justice to treatment of Arterial ulcers which are the most common ulcers seen in our practices.	s. We have reported the findings from our review of RCTs. We highlight findings (both positive and negative) where data support strong evidence to affect practice and policy. We agree that it is important to highlight positive findings if there is at least moderate certainty of benefit. However, it is also important to note areas where treatments are not effective or there is insufficient evidence, so that clinicians and patients can avoid use of treatments of low value/low effectiveness. We recognize that all patients have unique clinical circumstances–this is not unique to patients with chronic wound care needs. As with any condition, intervention, and outcome we summarize the findings from the available evidence, rate the quality of individual studies, determine strength of evidence, and make comments about the broader applicability to patients typically seen. Based on this evidence clinicians can make judgments regarding extrapolation to individual patients though we suggest that our findings can serve as the foundation for implementation.
s. Page 10 Discussion – In your discussion, please focus on positive findings. The studies may be of poor or moderate quality as such studies are often difficult to do. Please remember (and emphasize in your paper) that there are many reasons and factors affecting the occurrence of a wound, the needed treatment and the effectiveness of therapy. Each wound is different as it is the patient who owns the wound! That is not what was concluded previously in the previous pages!!	t. We have clarified that far fewer of the studies eligible for our review included an advanced therapy comparator.
t. Page 10 – "No treatment produced greater healing when compared to another advanced therapy." This statement is inaccurate! I do not believe that many of the studies (except a handful) compared one advanced therapy against another!	u. We have clarified this section. Overall the findings were mixed for each product group but there were some individual trials with positive results.
u. Page 11 Paragraph beginning with "The findings for venous ulcers .. silver products (that is not what was concluded previously in the previous pages!!), electromagnetic therapy (this contradicts what was concluded previously in the previous pages!!), significantly better healing (really? How come this was not noted in the sections above?)	v. We have clarified that the patients had undergone revascularization.
v. Page 11 Paragraph beginning with "We identified only one study of .... " Were these ulcers revascularized before use of apligraf or were they all ischemic wounds???	w. We have clarified ulcer location for studies cited throughout the report.
w. Main Report – Venous Leg Ulcer Description (70-90% of leg ulcers) – NOT foot ulcers! Location makes a huge difference on the etiology of the ulcer!	x. The literature typically refers to arterial ulcers as a group in the lower extremity. It does not tease out foot vs. leg. We agree that there are different factors involved in healing of the foot vs. the leg. We have clarified ulcer location for studies cited throughout the report.
x. Main Report – Arterial Leg Ulcer Description (6-10% of lower extremity ulcers) - Do these include ulcers in the foot? Or is it all in the leg. Please note, there is an anatomical difference when you talk about lower extremity, leg, or foot. Having said that you cannot combine the wound healing rate and success (or failure of) for all of these regions as each region heals differently?	y. The topic nominators requested that we include topical oxygen but no studies met our inclusion criteria. We have noted that in the report.
y. Main Report – Topical Oxygen Therapy Description – Is this even discussed in the above reported studies?	

Advanced Wound Care Therapies for Non-Healing Diabetic, Venous, and Arterial Ulcers: A Systematic Review

REVIEWER COMMENT	RESPONSE
The report and tables are comprehensive but limitations to the methodology are not highlighted in test. For example, recurrence of ulceration (or amputation) are usually lacking. Additionally, whether or not compliance with standard wound healing practices,(debridement, off-loading) is equally allocated between treatment and control groups is not highlighted.	We reported recurrence and amputation if reported by the study authors.

We have added comments about compliance. Most studies indicated that off loading etc. was part of the treatment protocol but few reported compliance measures (for treatment or control groups). |
| 1. As expected the results of the synthesis confirms the paucity of high level evidence to support the products used every day. The recommendations for criteria for future research are appreciated and will require that publications from this review be developed to get that word out.

2. Although the draft does speak somewhat to the limitations of the study I would recommend that it be highlighted and more specific to include important outcomes such as quality of life, recurrence, and prevention of amputations. | 1. Thank you
2. We have added more specific information to the limitations and future research sections. |
| 1. None of the citations described on page 77 have accompanying references.
2. In paragraph 3 of the discussion on page 77, greater emphasis should be placed the importance of offloading and adherence for DFU healing. The largest effect sizes for DFU healing in the literature are in offloading [1-3] causing leaders to suggest changes to the methodology for DFU trials.[4] This limitation should also be described on page 26 in the quality assessment section. Greater emphasis should also be placed on the importance of compression with VLU trials.[5]
3. The limitations and recommendations section do not adequately convey the magnitude of the problem associated with current industry sponsored trials' DFU inclusion/exclusion criteria. For example, ischemia and infection are either excluded or causes for censoring in DFU trials despite being highly prevalent conditions in clinical practice. For example, large cohort studies suggested a prevalence of clinically infected DFU's in 58-61% of patients [6, 7]; with up to 49% having peripheral arterial disease.[7] Fife also reports other populations that are excluded, including diabetes and significant comorbidities such as renal failure, ischemia, sickle cell, tobacco abuse, and steroid dependency [8] that are frequently encountered in practice.
4. In the executive summary, please provide point estimates for effect sizes in the silver, NPWT, and HBOT paragraphs on page 5. | 1. The reference list is now complete.
2. We have added information about off-loading for DFU healing and compression for VLU (including the suggested references). Thank you for the reference suggestions.
3. We have added to these sections. Thank you for the reference suggestions.
4. We have added absolute risk reduction data to the executive summary. |

REVIEWER COMMENT	RESPONSE
1. Armstrong, D.G., et al., Evaluation of Removable and Irremovable Cast Walkers in the Healing of Diabetic Foot Wounds: a Randomized Controlled Trial. Diabetes Care, 2005. 28(3): p. 551-4. 2. Armstrong, D.G., et al., Off-loading the diabetic foot wound: a randomized clinical trial. Diabetes Care, 2001. 24(6): p. 1019-22. 3. Katz, I.A., et al., A randomized trial of two irremovable off-loading devices in the management of plantar neuropathic diabetic foot ulcers. Diabetes Care, 2005. 28(3): p. 555-9. 4. Boulton, A.J. and D.G. Armstrong, Trials in neuropathic diabetic foot ulceration: time for a paradigm shift? Diabetes Care, 2003. 26(9): p. 2689-90. 5. Mustoe, T.A., K. O'Shaughnessy, and O. Kloeters, Chronic wound pathogenesis and current treatment strategies: a unifying hypothesis. Plast Reconstr Surg, 2006. 117(7 Suppl): p. 35S-41S. 6. Lavery, L.A., et al., Validation of the Infectious Diseases Society of America's diabetic foot infection classification system. Clin Infect Dis, 2007. 44(4): p. 562-5. 7. Prompers, L., et al., High prevalence of ischaemia, infection and serious comorbidity in patients with diabetic foot disease in Europe. Baseline results from the Eurodiale study. Diabetologia, 2007. 50(1): p. 18-25. 8. Fife, C., Wound Care in the 21st Century. US Surgery, 2007: p. 63-64.	
I personally found the information related to biological skin equivalents to be most interesting. These treatment adjuncts are VERY expensive and it would appear from the report that they offer only modest benefit in wound healing compared to standard therapy and no significant improvement in shortening the time for ulcer healing. My "take home" message here was that these products should be used very judiciously, if at all.	Thank you.
5. Are there any clinical performance measures, programs, quality improvement measures, patient care services, or conferences that will be directly affected by this report? If so, please provide detail.	Thank you – we will share these suggestions with the people responsible for dissemination of the report.
Yes. The wound clinics, podiatry sections, and possibly plastic surgery and general surgery sections if they deal with lower extremity wound care.	
Will likely impact criteria for use	
Yes, as stated above this synthesis will help us develop a guideline for the appropriate use of these expensive products using a combination of common sense and the evidence found in this study. We will have to resist the temptation to ban the use of products altogether but rather to place limits on how and where they are used. We must preserve the clinician's right to practice the art of medicine while recognizing we cannot continue to waste dollars on therapies that do not work. One telling point was that despite healing a wound faster or more completely there was no difference in all-cause mortality. This speaks to the need to develop algorithms that are interdisciplinary and address the systemic diseases as well as the wound.	

Advanced Wound Care Therapies for Non-Healing Diabetic,
Venous, and Arterial Ulcers: A Systematic Review

Evidence-based Synthesis Program

REVIEWER COMMENT	RESPONSE
This report has implications for National VA programs such as PACT and NSQIP. Results should be disseminated and presented at the VA's Annual Desert Foot Conference and HSR&D meeting. National presentations should also be considered at ADA and SAWC. The National PACT program may choose to study current use of advanced modality care in each strata using wound healing cameras to measure wound healing rates and appropriate use criteria and their effect on patient outcome in a pre & post-design.	
I would hope that the use of collagen products, biological dressings and platelet rich plasma would, for the most part, cease in most clinics treating the wounds described in the studies. On the other hand, the values of negative pressure wound therapy and hyperbaric oxygen in helping with wound healing in selected cases supports my own clinical experience in this area.	
6. Please provide any recommendations on how this report can be revised to more directly address or assist implementation needs.	
I worry that efficacy assessments do not always translate to general care of the VA	We appreciate this concern and have added the following statement to the discussion: "Our review assessed results from randomized controlled trials in selected populations and controlled settings. It is not well known how outcomes reported in these studies will translate to findings in daily practice settings including in Veterans Health Administration facilities. Patients were likely more compliant than typical patients and received very close monitoring. Therefore, results from these may overestimate benefits and underestimate harms in nonstudy populations."
You need to notify Dr. Jeff Robbins, the Chief of Podiatry at the VA central office about this report. He has a list of whom are most expert in the field within the VA. As there is a number of factors in treating wounds, the paper must emphasize the difficulty in performing studies and coming up with a conclusion on what is best for healing chronic wounds. The factors affecting doing a solid, strong study include but not limited to: the type of the wound, the host barriers, the host's associated comorbidities, the host's associated level of nutritional status, compliance with treatment, location of ulcers (plantar vs. dorsal), degree of blood flow (not all small vessel disease act the same!), the host's medications, …	We thank the reviewer for these comments. Dr. Robbins is involved with this project.
1) This is a long report and while the tables and appendices are important they should probably come at the end and be referenced in the body of the document. 2) We could release the executive summary widely and reference the full document. I am concerned that the field clinicians will not read a 178 page document. 3) In addition I am interested in helping in the production of some publications based on these findings to share with the scientific community.	1 and 2) We recognize the length of the report. We believe the information included is needed to provide the "interested reader" the full body of evidence we considered. We agree clinicians and policy makers are unlikely to read the whole document. We have tried to highlight the main findings in the executive summary and are willing to conduct other dissemination activities including Cyberseminars, Management Briefs etc. to further convey the main messages to a wide audience. 3) We are considering derivative manuscripts from this report.
There is a growing chasm between operations and research. Those who conduct systematic reviews or meta-analyses frequently are not PI's conducting the studies or actively engaged in patient care.[1] A careful compilation of improvement opportunities for study designs should be created for both funding agencies (including industry) and PI's. These should also be disseminated to NIH and VA program officers. 1. Gottrup, F., Controversies in performing a randomized control trial and a systemic review. Wound Repair Regen, 2012. 20(4): p. 447-8.	We have cited several documents detailing recommendations for future research.
The report is extremely well done and readable as it stands. I have no recommendations for improvement.	Thank you.

111

APPENDIX D. EVIDENCE TABLES

Table 1. Study Characteristics Table

Study, Year Country Funding Source	Inclusion/Exclusion Criteria	Patient Characteristics Ulcer Type	Intervention Comparator Length of Follow-up	Study Quality
Abidia 2003[49] United Kingdom Funding Source: NR Therapy Type: Hyperbaric oxygen (HBOT)	Inclusion: diabetes; ischemic lower extremity ulcers (>1 cm and <10 cm in maximum diameter); no signs of healing for >6 weeks despite optimum medical management; occlusive arterial disease confirmed by ankle-brachial pressure index <0.8 (or great toe <0.7 if calf vessels incompressible) Exclusion: planned vascular surgery, angioplasty, or thrombolysis	N=16 (of 18 randomized) Age (years): 71 Gender (% male): 50 Race/ethnicity: NR BMI: NR Pre-albumin: NR HbA,c (%): NR Smoking: 19% # Work days missed: NR ABI: <0.8 for inclusion Wound location: foot Wound type: ischemic diabetic Wound size, mm^2 (median): HBOT 106; control 78 Wound grade (Wagner*, %): Grade I 6; II 94 Wound duration, months: HBOT 6; control 9 Comorbid conditions (%): History of CAD/CVD: (previous bypass 31, angioplasty 6) History of DM: 100 History of amputation: minor 19	Intervention (n=9): HBOT; 2.4 ATA for 90 minutes on 30 occasions over 6 weeks; multi-place chamber Control (n=9): sham (hyperbaric air) ALL: specialized multidisciplinary wound management program (off-loading, debridement, moist dressing) *Antibiotic Use:* As needed *Treatment Duration:* 6 weeks *Follow-up Duration:* 1 year *Study Withdrawal (%):* 20 (n=2) *Treatment Compliance:* "The protocol was strictly followed throughout the study"	Allocation concealment: Adequate Blinding: Patients, investigators, outcome assessors Intention to treat analysis (ITT): No, two withdrawals not included in analysis Withdrawals/dropouts adequately described: Yes

Study, Year Country Funding Source	Inclusion/Exclusion Criteria	Patient Characteristics Ulcer Type	Intervention Comparator Length of Follow-up	Study Quality
Agrawal 2009[28] India Funding Source: NR Therapy Type: Platelet-derived Growth Factor	Inclusion: ≥30 years of age; Wagner stage I, II, III, or IV ulcers; foot ulcer duration >3 months; free of infection; adequate lower-limb blood supply (transcutaneous oxygen tension ≥30 mmHg); no or moderate peripheral vascular disease Exclusion: active neoplastic disease; diagnosis of active infection characterized by warmth, erythema, lymphangitis, lymphadenopathy, oedema, or pain; received immunosuppressive therapy during the preceding three months; liver disease, pulmonary tuberculosis, thyroid disorder uremia, alcoholism or renal insufficiency; undergoing vascular reconstruction or receiving steroid or anticoagulant therapy	N=28 Age (years): 55 Gender (% male): 68 Race/ethnicity: NR BMI: 25.7 Pre-albumin: NR HbA$_1$c (%): 8.8 Smoking: NR # Work days missed: NR ABI: NR Wound location: foot Wound type: diabetic Wound size: 41.5 cm^2 (ulcer size significantly larger in study group p=0.003) Wound grade: NR Wound duration: NR Infection: excluded Comorbid conditions (%): Diabetes: 100	Intervention (n=14): rhPDGF 0.01% gel at 2.2ug/cm^2/day Comparator (n=14): placebo gel at 2.2ug/cm^2/day ALL: standard regimen of high-quality care (included glycemic control, debridement, dressings, pressure relief) *Antibiotic Use:* as needed *Treatment Duration:* 12 weeks *Follow-up Duration:* NR *Study Withdrawal (%):* 18 (all from control group at week 12) *Treatment Compliance:* NR	Allocation concealment: Unclear Blinding: Unclear Intention to treat analysis (ITT): No Withdrawals/dropouts adequately described: Partial – 5 withdrawals from the control group with no reason for withdrawal
Aminian 2000[27] Iran Funding Source: Government Therapy Type: Platelet-Derived Growth Factor	Inclusion: chronic non-healing diabetic ulcers of at least eight weeks duration; controlled blood sugar; normal peripheral blood platelet count (>150,000/cu mm); negative history of malignancy Exclusion: determined to have non-diabetic ulcers	N=12 ulcers (7 patients) of 14 ulcers (9 patients) randomized Age (years): 60 Gender (% male): 100 Race/ethnicity: NR BMI: NR Pre-albumin: NR HbA$_1$c (%): NR Smoking: NR # Work days missed: NR ABI: NR Wound location: foot Wound type: diabetic ulcer Wound size: 5.9 cm^2 Wound grade: NR Wound duration: 12.9 wks Infection: NR Comorbid conditions (%): Diabetes: 100	Intervention (n=7 ulcers): autologous platelet extract (APE) + silver sulfadiazine dressing 12 hours on and 12 hours off Comparator (n=5 ulcers): saline solution and silver sulfadiazine 12 hours on and 12 hours off ALL: supportive, conventional care (debridement, blood sugar checked weekly, off-loading) *Antibiotic Use:* oral, if needed *Treatment Duration:* 8 weeks *Follow-up Duration:* NR *Study Withdrawal (%):* 22% *Treatment Compliance:* 1/9 pts withdrawn for non-compliance	Allocation concealment: Inadequate Blinding: Unclear Intention to treat analysis (ITT): No Withdrawals/dropouts adequately described: Yes – 2 patients with 2 ulcers excluded after entering study (non-compliance, non-diabetic ulcer)

113

Study, Year Country Funding Source	Inclusion/Exclusion Criteria	Patient Characteristics Ulcer Type	Intervention Comparator Length of Follow-up	Study Quality
Armstrong 2005[81] Apelqvist 2008[82] United States (18 sites) Funding Source: Industry (not involved in analysis or write-up of manuscript; did not maintain veto power over final article) Therapy Type: Negative Pressure Wound Therapy	Inclusion: age ≥18; wound from diabetic foot amputation to transmetatarsal level of foot; evidence of adequate perfusion (transcutaneous O2 on dorsum of foot ≥30 mmHg or ABI ≥0.7 and ≤1.2, and toe pressure ≥30 mmHg); University of Texas grade 2 or 3 in depth Exclusion: active Charcot arthropathy of foot; wound from burn, venous insufficiency, untreated cellulitis or osteomyelitis, collagen vascular disease, malignant disease, or uncontrolled hyperglycemia (HbA$_1$c >12%); treated with corticosteroids, immunosuppressive drugs, or chemotherapy; VAC therapy in past 30 days, present or previous (past 30 days) treatment with growth factors; normothermic therapy, hyperbaric medicine, or bioengineered tissue	N=162 Age (years): 59 Gender (% male): 81 Race/ethnicity (%): Non-Hispanic white: 48; African-American: 17; Mexican-American: 32; Native American: 3 BMI: 31 Pre-albumin (g/L): 0.19 HbA$_1$c (%): 8.2 Smoking: 9% # Work days missed: NR ABI: 1.1 Wound location: foot Wound type: amputation Wound size: 20.7 cm^2 Wound grade: U of Texas 2/3 Wound duration: 1.5 months Comorbid conditions (%): History of DM: 100 (90% T2)	Intervention (n=77): VAC system; dressing changes every 48 hrs Comparator (n=85): standard care (moist wound therapy with alginates, hydrocolloids, foams, or hydrogels; dressing changes every day unless otherwise advised ALL: off-loading therapy as indicated; sharp debridement at randomization and as needed *Antibiotic Use:* NR *Treatment Duration:* wound closure or 112 days *Follow-up Duration:* none *Study Withdrawal (%):* 0 *Treatment Compliance:* NR	Allocation concealment: Adequate Blinding: Partial (independently assessed and confirmed closure with digital planimetry) Intention to treat analysis (ITT): Yes – no withdrawals Withdrawals/dropouts adequately described: Yes – no withdrawals
Belcaro 2010[38] Italy Funding Source: NR Therapy Type: Silver Oxide Ointment	Inclusion: *Venous Ulcer (VU) Patients:* chronic venous ulcers, venous microangiopathy, and perimalleaolar ulcerations *Diabetic Ulcer (DU) Patients:* diabetic microangiopathy and plantar ulcers due to reduced arterial pressure, diabetic microangiopahty and neuropathy, and localized infection Exclusion: *Venous Ulcer Patients:* venous thrombosis or arterial problems in past year; severe ischemia and necrosis (based on Doppler detected tibial pulse) *Diabetic Ulcer Patients:* none reported	*Venous Ulcer Patients:* N=82 Age (years): 47 Gender (% male): 46 *Diabetic Ulcer Patients:* N=66 Age (years): 55.9 Gender (% male): 44 *Both Groups:* Race/ethnicity: NR BMI: NR Pre-albumin: NR HbA$_1$c (%): NR Smoking: NR # Work days missed: NR ABI: NR Wound location: plantar (DU) Wound type: venous, diabetic Wound size: VU 3.2 cm^2, DU 2.2 cm^2 Wound grade: NR Wound duration: NR Comorbid conditions (%): NR	Intervention (n=44 VU, n=34 DU): silver ointment around and at edges of ulcerated area twice daily after noninvasive washing; bandage and elastic stocking Comparator (n=38 VU, n=32 DU): cleansing & wound care; compression (mild for DU) *Antibiotic Use:* NR *Treatment Duration:* 4 weeks *Follow-up Duration:* No follow-up post tx *Study Withdrawal (%):* 0 *Treatment Compliance:* NR	Allocation concealment: Unclear Blinding: Unclear Intention to treat analysis (ITT): Yes (no withdrawals) Withdrawals/dropouts adequately described: Yes (none)

Advanced Wound Care Therapies for Non-Healing Diabetic, Venous, and Arterial Ulcers: A Systematic Review

Study, Year Country Funding Source	Inclusion/Exclusion Criteria	Patient Characteristics Ulcer Type	Intervention Comparator Length of Follow-up	Study Quality
Bhansali 2009[30] India Funding Source: Industry (provided gel) Therapy Type: Platelet-derived Growth Factor	Inclusion: >20 years old with type 1 or 2 diabetes; at least one neuropathic plantar ulcer of Wagner grade ≥ 2 without X-ray evidence of osteomyelitis; ABI>0.9; controlled infection after run-in Exclusion: none reported	N=20 (24 ulcers) Age (years): 51 Gender (% male): 60 Race/ethnicity: NR BMI: 24 Pre-albumin: NR HbA$_1$c (%): 8.1 Smoking: NR # Work days missed: NR ABI: 1.05 Wound location: forefoot: 75%; mid: 20%; hind: 5% Wound type: diabetic Wound size: 14.6 cm^2 Wound grade: Wagner ≥ 2 Wound duration: <4 weeks=20%; >4 weeks=80% Infection: 45% Comorbid conditions (%): History of DM: 100% History of amputation: 35%	Intervention (n=13): 0.01% rh-PDGF-BB gel Comparator (n=11): standard wound care (saline soaked dressing) ALL: daily dressing changes; off-loading (85% total contact cast, 10% bedridden, 5% special shoe) *Antibiotic Use:* As needed *Treatment Duration:* 20 weeks *Follow-up Duration:* NR *Study Withdrawal (%):* 0 *Treatment Compliance:* NR	Allocation concealment: Unclear Blinding: No (open label) Intention to treat analysis (ITT): Yes Withdrawals/dropouts adequately described: Yes (none)
Bishop 1992[63] United States (2 sites) Funding Source: Industry Therapy Type: Silver Products	Inclusion: age 21 to 90 years; venous stasis ulcers of at least 3 months duration; surface area 3 cm^2 to 50 cm^2; negative pregnancy test and using adequate contraceptive (women of childbearing age) Exclusion: hypersensitivity to any components of test medication; >10^5 bacteria/gram of tissue in the ulcer; systemic sepsis or presence of bone infection; ABI<0.5; hypercupremia (Wilson's disease); systemic immunosuppressive or cytotoxic therapy; insulin-dependent diabetes mellitus	N=86 (of 93 randomized) Age (years): 56 Gender (% male): 50 Race/ethnicity: white: 62; black: 33; other: 6 BMI: NR Pre-albumin: NR HbA$_1$c (%): NR Smoking: 33.7% currently # Work days missed: NR ABI: NR Wound location: "lower extremity" Wound type: venous stasis Wound size: 10.5 cm^2 Wound grade: NR Wound duration: 46.4 months Comorbid conditions (%): History of DM: 9%	Intervention (n=29): 0.4% tripeptide copper complex cream Comparator (n=28): 1% silver sulphadiazine cream Placebo (n=29): tripeptide vehicle ALL: applied daily following saline rinse; non-adherent dressing and elastic wrap; limb elevated when sitting; no standing >2 hrs *Antibiotic Use:* NR *Treatment Duration:* 4 weeks *Follow-up Duration:* 1 year *Study Withdrawal (%):* 7.5 *Treatment Compliance:* patient diary and medication weighed at end of study; results NR	Allocation concealment: Unclear Blinding: Yes (evaluator) Intention to treat analysis (ITT): No Withdrawals/dropouts adequately described: Partial (3 were immediate dropouts; 4 additional patients did not complete the trial; reasons not provided)

Advanced Wound Care Therapies for Non-Healing Diabetic, Venous, and Arterial Ulcers: A Systematic Review

Study, Year Country Funding Source	Inclusion/Exclusion Criteria	Patient Characteristics Ulcer Type	Intervention Comparator Length of Follow-up	Study Quality
Blair 1988[64] United Kingdom Funding Source: NR Therapy Type: Silver Products	Inclusion: ulcers up to 10 cm² Exclusion: ABI<0.8	N=60 Age (years): 69 Gender (% male): NR Race/ethnicity: NR BMI: NR Pre-albumin: NR HbA₁c (%): NR Smoking: NR # Work days missed: NR ABI: NR Wound location: NR Wound type: venous Wound size: 3.4 cm² Wound grade: NR Wound duration: 26.2 months since ulcer was last healed Comorbid conditions (%): NR	Intervention (n=30): silver sulphadiazine dressing (Flamazine) Comparator (n=30): non-adherent and non-occlusive dressing ALL: out-patient treatment; dressings changed weekly in venous ulcer clinic; standard high pressure graduated compression bandage over the dressing *Antibiotic Use:* NR *Treatment Duration:* 12 weeks *Follow-up Duration:* none *Study Withdrawal (%):* 7% *Treatment Compliance:* NR	Allocation concealment: Adequate Blinding: Unclear Intention to treat analysis (ITT): Yes Withdrawals/dropouts adequately described: Yes
Blume 2008[42] United States and Canada (29 sites) Funding Source: Industry Therapy Type: Negative Pressure Wound Therapy	Inclusion: diabetic adults (18+); stage 2 or 3 (Wagner's) calcaneal, dorsal, or plantar foot ulcer; ≥2 cm² after debridement; adequate blood circulation (dorsum transcutaneous O₂ test ≥30 mmHg; ABI 0.7-1.2 with toe pressure ≥30 mmHg) or triphasic or biphasic Doppler waveforms at ankle Exclusion: active Charcot disease; electrical, chemical, or radiation burns; collagen vascular disease; ulcer malignancy; untreated osteomyelitis; cellulitis; uncontrolled hyperglycemia; inadequate lower extremity perfusion; normothermic or hyperbaric oxygen therapy; use of corticosteroids, immunosupressants, or chemotherapy; growth factor products; skin or dermal substitutes within 30 days; enzymatic debridement; pregnant or nursing	N=335 (of 341 randomized) Age (years): 59 Gender (% male): 78 Race/ethnicity (%): African-American: 15; Caucasian: 58; Hispanic: 24; Native American: 2; other: 1 BMI: NR Pre-albumin: 20.5 HbA₁c (%): 8.2 Smoking: 19% # Work days missed: NR ABI: 1.0 Wound location: calcaneal, dorsal, or plantar Wound type: diabetic ulcer Wound size: 12.3 cm² Wound grade: 2 or 3 Wound duration: 202 days Comorbid conditions (%): History of DM: 100	Intervention (n=172): NPWT - vacuum-assisted closure therapy; dressing changes every 48-72 hrs Comparator (n=169): advanced moist wound therapy (AMWT) Off-load: NPWT 97%; AMWT 98% *Antibiotic Use:* NR (28% treated for infection before randomization) *Treatment Duration:* 112 days *Follow-up Duration:* 3 and 9 months after closure *Study Withdrawal (%):* NPWT: 32%; AMWT: 25% *Treatment Compliance:* 6/169 (4%) in NPWT group were non-compliant vs. 0% in AMWT group (not defined)	Allocation concealment: Adequate Blinding: Patients and physicians not blinded; unclear if outcome assessment was blinded Intention to treat analysis (ITT): Modified (received at least one post-baseline treatment) Withdrawals/dropouts adequately described: Yes

Advanced Wound Care Therapies for Non-Healing Diabetic, Venous, and Arterial Ulcers: A Systematic Review

Study, Year Country Funding Source	Inclusion/Exclusion Criteria	Patient Characteristics Ulcer Type	Intervention Comparator Length of Follow-up	Study Quality
Blume 2011[15] United States (22 sites) Funding Source: Industry Therapy Type: Collagen	Inclusion: type 1 or 2 diabetes; over age 18 yrs; Wagner Grade 1 cutaneous lower extremity ulcer, 1.5-10.0 cm^2; present ≥6 wks; peripheral neuropathy; adequate blood flow (TcpO$_2$ >40mmHg or toe pressure ≥40mmHg) Exclusion: HbA$_1$c >12%; ulcer on heel; cellulitis; biopsy positive for beta hemolytic streptococci or total bacterial load >1X10^6 CFU/g; decrease in ulcer size >30% from screening to Tx day 1	N=52 Age (years): 56 Gender (% male): 77 Race/ethnicity (%): white 64, black 12, Hispanic 23, other 2 BMI: 34 Pre-albumin: NR HbA$_1$c (%): 8.0 Smoking: NR # Work days missed: NR ABI: NR Wound location: 89% plantar Wound type: diabetic Wound size: 2.9 cm^2 Wound duration: 15.1 months Comorbid conditions (%): History of DM: 100	Intervention (n=33): formulated collagen gel (FCG) (combined 1 dose and 2 dose groups) (NOTE: included 2nd intervention arm with non-FDA product) Comparator (n=19): standard care (debride, moist dressing) ALL: debridement; 2 wk standard care run-in; off-loading shoe *Antibiotic Use:* NR *Treatment Duration:* 12 weeks *Follow-up Duration:* None *Study Withdrawal (%):* 6/5 (8/124) *Treatment Compliance:* see WD	Allocation concealment: Unclear Blinding: Investigators were blinded; other study personnel were not Intention to treat analysis (ITT): Yes for safety analysis; per-protocol for other outcomes Withdrawals/dropouts adequately described: Yes (including 2 in FCG group for non-compliance)
Brigido 2006[74] United States Funding Source: NR Therapy Type: Collagen	Inclusion: full thickness (Wagner grade II) chronic wound ≥6 weeks without epidermal coverage; non-infected; palpable/ audible pulse to the lower extremity Exclusion: none reported	N=28 Age (years): 64 Gender (% male): NR Race/ethnicity: NR BMI: NR Pre-albumin: NR HbA$_1$c (%): 8.0 Smoking: NR # Work days missed: NR ABI: NR Wound location: leg/foot Wound type: mixed Wound size: NR Wound grade: Wagner grade II Wound duration: NR Infection: excluded if infected Comorbid conditions (%): NR	Intervention (n=14): Graftjacket (single application); mineral oil soaked fluff compression dressing changed on days 5, 10, and 15 then weekly assessment Comparator (n=14): Curasol wound gel; gauze dressing; weekly debridement ALL: initial sharp debridement; off-loading with walking boot *Antibiotic Use:* NR *Treatment Duration:* 16 weeks *Follow-up Duration:* None *Study Withdrawal (%):* 0 *Treatment Compliance:* NR	Allocation concealment: Unclear Blinding: No Intention to treat analysis (ITT): Yes Withdrawals/dropouts adequately described: Yes – all patients completed study

117

Study, Year Country Funding Source	Inclusion/Exclusion Criteria	Patient Characteristics Ulcer Type	Intervention Comparator Length of Follow-up	Study Quality
Chang 2000[73] United States Funding Source: NR Therapy Type: Biological Skin Equivalent	Inclusion: non-healing foot ulcer or required partial open foot amputation; ABI <0.5 prior to revascularization surgery; underwent bypass or angioplasty within 60 days of inclusion Exclusion: ABI <0.7 after revascularization surgery; recent steroid use; chemotherapy; previous radiation; wound <2.0 cm²; infected wound, necrotic tissue, exposed bone, or exposed tendons	N=31 Age (years): 70 Gender (% male): 77 Race/ethnicity (%): NR BMI: NR HbA₁c (%): NR Smoking: NR # Work days missed: NR ABI: NR (see inclusion criteria) Wound type: previously ischemic wounds s/p revascularization surgery Wound size: 4.8 cm² Wound duration: NR Infection: excluded Comorbid conditions (%): History of DM: 58% History of amputation: 45% History of PVD: 100% History of renal failure: 39%	Intervention (n=21): meshed (N=10) or unmeshed (N=11) tissue graft (Apligraf): non-adherent dressing, Unna boot & ace wrap; followed every 5-7 days (or more) for 1st month; Unna boot dressing changes each visit until graft maturation Comparator (n=10): moist saline gauze sponges with dry cotton gauze wrapping; changed 2x/day *Antibiotic Use:* NR *Treatment Duration:* wound closure or ≥ 6 months after randomization *Follow-up Duration:* same *Study Withdrawal (%):* NR *Treatment Compliance:* NR	Allocation concealment: Unclear Blinding: No Intention to treat analysis (ITT): Unclear Withdrawals/dropouts adequately described: Unclear if any dropouts
d'Hemecourt 1998[35] United States (10 sites) Funding Source: Industry Therapy Type: Platelet-derived Growth Factors	Inclusion: ≥19 years old; type 1 or 2 diabetes; at least one full thickness (Stage 3 or 4) diabetic ulcer of >8 weeks duration; wound size 1.0-10.0 cm²; adequate arterial circulation Exclusion: osteomyelitis affecting target ulcer area; >3 chronic ulcers present at baseline; non-diabetic wounds; cancer at time of enrollment; use of concomitant medications (corticosteroids, chemotherapy, immunosuppressive agents); pregnant or nursing	N=172 Age (years): 58 Gender (% male): 74 Race/ethnicity (%): white: 85; black: 10; other: 5 BMI: NR Pre-albumin: NR HbA₁c (%): NR Smoking: NR # Work days missed: NR ABI: NR Wound location: right leg: 3%; left leg: 4%; right foot: 47%; left foot: 47% Wound type: diabetic ulcer Wound size: 3.2 cm² Wound grade: 97% Stage III Wound duration: 42.3 weeks Infection: NR Comorbid conditions (%): Diabetes: 100	Intervention (n=30): becaplermin gel 100ug/g and standard care Comparator A (n=70): sodium carboxymethylcellulose Gel (NaCMC) and standard care Comparator B (n=68): standard care – sharp debridement, saline gauze dressing changes every 12 hours, off-loading *Antibiotic Use:* systemic control of infection if present *Treatment Duration:* 20 weeks *Follow-up Duration:* NR *Study Withdrawal (%):* 24 *Treatment Compliance:* NR	Allocation concealment: Unclear Blinding: Yes – patients, evaluators Intention to treat analysis (ITT): Yes Withdrawals/dropouts adequately described: Yes

Study, Year Country Funding Source	Inclusion/Exclusion Criteria	Patient Characteristics Ulcer Type	Intervention Comparator Length of Follow-up	Study Quality
DiDomenico 2011[26] United States Funding Source: Industry Therapy Type: Biological Skin Equivalent	Inclusion: type 1 or 2 diabetes; Wagner grade 1 or University of Texas 1a ulcer; wound duration >4 weeks; area 0.5-4 cm^2; HbA$_1$c <12; ABI >0.75; palpable pulses on the study foot; able to comply with off-loading

Exclusion: infection or gangrenous tissue or abscesses; exposed bone, tendon, or joint capsule; non-diabetic etiology; use of topical medications that may affect graft material; adjuvant therapy such as hyperbaric oxygen; wound depth <9 mm | N=28 patients (29 wounds) Age (years): NR Gender (% male): NR Race/ethnicity: NR BMI: NR Pre-albumin: NR HbA$_1$c (%): NR Smoking: NR # Work days missed: NR ABI: NR Wound location: NR Wound type: diabetic ulcer Wound size: 1.9 cm^2 Wound grade: see inclusion Wound duration: see inclusion Comorbid conditions (%): NR | Intervention (n=17 wounds): Apligraf; up to 5 applications Comparator (n=12 wounds): Theraskin; up to 5 applications ALL: debridement, off-loading; dressing changes every other day or daily, as needed Antibiotic Use: NR Treatment Duration: 12 weeks Follow-up Duration: to 20 weeks Study Withdrawal (%): NR Treatment Compliance: NR | Allocation concealment: Unclear Blinding: Unclear Intention to treat analysis (ITT): Unclear Withdrawals/dropouts adequately described: Yes |
| Dimakakos 2009[65] Greece Funding Source: NR Therapy Type: Silver Dressing | Inclusion: leg ulcer classified as exclusively infected and venous in origin Exclusion: pregnancy; psychiatric disorders; diabetes; collagen disease; steroid use; history of allergies; ABPI<1 | N=42 Age (years): 60 Gender (% male): 38 Race/ethnicity: NR BMI: NR Pre-albumin: NR HbA$_1$c (%): NR Smoking: NR # Work days missed: NR ABI: NR Wound location: leg Wound type: venous Wound size: NR Wound grade: NR Wound duration: 62% >1 mo Infection: excluded Comorbid conditions: 0% DM | Intervention (n=21): non-adhesive silver-releasing foam Comparator (n=21): non-adhesive foam ALL: cleansing with sterile water and 10% povidone iodine solution; compression bandage Antibiotic Use: as needed Treatment Duration: 9 weeks Follow-up Duration: NR Study Withdrawal (%): NR Treatment Compliance: NR | Allocation concealment: Unclear Blinding: Unclear Intention to treat analysis (ITT): No withdrawals/ dropouts reported Withdrawals/dropouts adequately described: None reported |

Advanced Wound Care Therapies for Non-Healing Diabetic, Venous, and Arterial Ulcers: A Systematic Review

Study, Year Country Funding Source	Inclusion/Exclusion Criteria	Patient Characteristics Ulcer Type	Intervention Comparator Length of Follow-up	Study Quality
Donaghue 1998[17] United States Funding Source: Industry Therapy Type: Collagen	Inclusion: >21 years of age; serum albumin >2.5 grams/dl; adequate blood flow to lower extremity (palpable pulses); foot ulceration of at least 1 cm^2 Exclusion: severe renal or liver impairment (liver or creatinine tests 2 or more times higher than normal); presence of any disorder that may interfere with wound healing; evidence of osteomyelitis; clinical signs of infection; history of drug or alcohol abuse	N=75 Age (years): 59 Gender (% male): 72 Race/ethnicity: NR BMI: NR Pre-albumin: 3.7 HbA$_1$c (%): NR Smoking: NR # Work days missed: NR ABI: NR Wound location: foot Wound type: diabetic ulcer Wound size: 2.7 cm^2 Wound grade: Wagner I: 12%; II: 75%; III: 13% Wound duration: 172 days Infection: excluded Comorbid conditions (%): Diabetes: 100	Intervention (n=50): collagen-alginate Comparator (n=25): conventional treatment with saline-moistened gauze ALL: felted foam dressing with window at site of ulcer; use of healing sandals; patient self dressing change as required *Antibiotic Use:* NR *Treatment Duration:* 8 weeks *Follow-up Duration:* NR *Study Withdrawal (%):* 19 *Treatment Compliance:* NR	Allocation concealment: Unclear Blinding: No Intention to treat analysis (ITT): Yes Withdrawals/dropouts adequately described: Yes
Driver 2006[37] United States (14 sites including VA wound care clinics) Funding Source: Industry Therapy Type: Platelet Rich Plasma	Inclusion: type 1 or 2 diabetes; age 18-95; ulcer >4 weeks; HbA$_1$c <12%; index ulcer on plantar, medial, or lateral foot; area 0.5-20 cm^2; Charcot deformity free of acute changes & undergone structural consolidation; ulcer free of infection; no bone, muscle, ligament, or tendon exposure; ≥4 cm from any other wound; adequate perfusion Exclusion: investigational drug or device trial (30 days); ulcer size decrease ≥50% in 7 day run-in; non-diabetic ulcers; serum albumin <2.5 g/dL; hemoglobin <10.5 mg/dL; radiation or chemotherapy; renal dialysis; immune deficiency; known abnormal platelet activation disorder; peripheral vascular repair in past 30 days; known or suspected osteomyelitis; surgery required for healing; exposed tendon, ligaments, muscle, or bone; disorder that may affect compliance; alcohol or drug abuse (past year)	N=40 (of 72 randomized) Age (years): 57 Gender (% male): 80 Race/ethnicity: Caucasian: 60; Hispanic: 30; black: 7.5; other: 2.5 BMI: NR Pre-albumin: NR HbA$_1$c (%): 7.9 Smoking: NR # Work days missed: NR ABI: NR Wound location (%): right foot: 60; left foot: 40; toe: 38; heel: 40 (NR for 9 patients) Wound type: diabetic ulcer Wound size: 3.5 cm^2 Wound grade: NR Wound duration: NR Infection: excluded Comorbid conditions (%): Diabetes: 100	Intervention (n=40): platelet rich plasma (AutoloGel); applied twice weekly Comparator (n=32): saline gel (Normlgel); applied twice weekly *Antibiotic Use:* NR *Treatment Duration:* 12 weeks *Follow-up Duration:* 3 months *Study Withdrawal (%):* 44 *Treatment Compliance:* NR	Allocation concealment: Adequate Blinding: Yes (patients, investigators, outcome assessors) Intention to treat analysis (ITT): Yes but focused on per protocol analysis due to protocol violations (n=24) and failure to complete treatment (n=8) Withdrawals/dropouts adequately described: Yes

Study, Year Country Funding Source	Inclusion/Exclusion Criteria	Patient Characteristics Ulcer Type	Intervention Comparator Length of Follow-up	Study Quality
Duzgun 2008[47] Turkey Funding Source: NR Therapy Type: Hyperbaric Oxygen (HBOT)	Inclusion: diabetic; ≥18 years; foot wound present for ≥4 weeks despite appropriate local and systemic wound care; wounds were categorized according to a modification of the Wagner classification; contraindication to hyperbaric oxygen therapy (untreated pneumothorax, COPD, history of otic surgery, upper respiratory tract infection, febrile state, history of idiopathic convulsion, hypoglycemia, current corticosteroid, amphetamine, catecholamine, or thyroid hormone use) Exclusion: none reported	N=100 Age (years): 61 Gender (% male): HBOT 74%; Std Care 54%; p<0.05 Race/ethnicity: NR BMI (>30, %): 63 (HBOT 80% Std Care 46%; p<0.05) Pre-albumin: NR HbA₁c (%): 8.4 Smoking: 56% # Work days missed: NR ABI: NR Wound location (%): foot Wound type: diabetic Wound size, cm²: NR Wound grade (Wagner) (%): Grade II 18%; III 37%; IV 45% Wound duration, months: NR Comorbid conditions (%): History of DM: 100% History of HTN: 60% History of hyperlipidemia: 58%	Intervention (n=50): HBOT administered at maximum working pressure of 20 ATA; unichamber pressure room; volume of 10m³ at 2 to 3 ATA for 90 minutes + standard therapy; treatment was 2 sessions/day, then 1 session on the following day Comparator (n=50): standard therapy ALL: daily wound care (dressing changes, debridement; amputation when indicated *Antibiotic Use:* as needed *Treatment Duration:* 20 to 30 days *Follow-up Duration:* 92 weeks *Study Withdrawal (%):* None reported *Treatment Compliance:* NR	Allocation concealment: Inadequate "according to a predetermined sequence wherein consecutively enrolled patients corresponding to an even random number received ST, and those corresponding to an odd random number received ST+HBOT" Blinding: None reported Intention to treat analysis (ITT): Yes Withdrawals/dropouts adequately described: None reported
Edmonds 2009[25] Europe, Australia (multi-site) Funding Source: NR Therapy Type: Biological Skin Equivalent	Inclusion: diabetes type 1 or 2; 18–80 years old; primarily neuropathic origin, not infected; present at least 2 weeks; surface area 1–16 cm²; adequate vascular supply; able to follow treatment protocol (incl. off-loading) Exclusion: active Charcot foot; non-neuropathic origin; target ulcer with evidence of skin cancer; osteomyelitis at any location requiring treatment; infected target ulcer; medical condition which could impair healing; pregnant; corticosteroid use (current or prior); use of immunosuppressive agents; radiation therapy or chemotherapy; prior treatment of study wound; history of drug or alcohol abuse (in past year)	N=72 (of 82 randomized) Age (years): 59 Gender (% male): 86 Race/ethnicity (%): NR BMI: NR HbA₁c (%): NR Smoking: NR # Work days missed: NR ABI: NR Wound location: plantar, forefoot Wound type: diabetic ulcer Wound size: 3.0 cm² Wound grade: NR Wound duration: 1.8 years Comorbid Conditions (%): Diabetes: 100	Intervention (n=33): Apligraf (at week 0 and weeks 4 and 8, if needed) + Mepitel contact layer dressing Comparator (n=39): Mepitel ALL: weekly debridement if needed; saline-moist dressing; off-loading *Antibiotic Use:* NR *Treatment Duration:* 12 weeks *Follow-up Duration:* 24 weeks post-treatment *Study Withdrawal (%):* 12 *Treatment Compliance:* NR	Allocation concealment: Adequate Blinding: No Intention to treat analysis (ITT): No Withdrawals/dropouts adequately described: Yes

Advanced Wound Care Therapies for Non-Healing Diabetic, Venous, and Arterial Ulcers: A Systematic Review

Study, Year Country Funding Source	Inclusion/Exclusion Criteria	Patient Characteristics Ulcer Type	Intervention Comparator Length of Follow-up	Study Quality
Falanga 1998[54] United States (15 sites) Funding Source: Industry Therapy Type: Biological Skin Equivalent	Inclusion:18-85 years of age; ulcer due to venous insufficiency (clinical signs/symptoms); no significant arterial insufficiency (ABI>0.65); evidence of venous insufficiency (air plethysmography or photo-plethysmography (refilling time <20 seconds) Exclusion: clinical signs of cellulitis, vasculitis, or collagen vascular disease; pregnancy or lactation; uncontrolled diabetes; other impaired wound healing (renal, hepatic, hematologic, neurologic, or immunological disease); received corticosteroids, immunosuppressive agents, radiation therapy, or chemotherapy in past month	N=275 (of 309 randomized) Age (years): 60 Gender (% male): 52 Race/ethnicity(%): white 76; black 18; Asian 1; Hispanic 4 BMI: NR HbA$_1$c (%): NR Smoking: NR # Work days missed: NR ABI: >0.65 per inclusion Wound location: NR Wound type: venous Wound size: 1.2 cm^2 Wound duration: <6 months: 31%; 6-12 months: 21%; 1-2 years: 14%; >2 years: 35% Comorbid conditions (%): NR	Intervention (n=146): human skin equivalent (Apligraf) + elastic wrap; applied up to 5 times in first 3 wks (days 0, 3-5, 7, 14, and/or 21) until estimated area of graft "take" >50%; compression alone continued for total of 8 wks Comparator (n=129): compression therapy reapplied weekly for 8 wks *Antibiotic Use:* NR *Treatment Duration:* 8 weeks *Follow-up Duration:* 6 months *Study Withdrawal (%):* unclear; analysis of 275/309 (89%) *Treatment Compliance:* NR	Allocation concealment: Adequate Blinding: No Intention to treat analysis (ITT): No Withdrawals/dropouts adequately described: Partial – number of dropouts (n=72) is different than number not included in data analysis (n=34)
Falanga 1999[55] See Falanga1998[54] United States (15 sites) Funding Source: Therapy Type: Biological Skin Equivalent	Inclusion: same as above with ulcer duration of >1 year Exclusion: same as above	N=120 for efficacy analysis (demographics from n=122; 2 extra in treatment group by "double randomization") Age (years): 58 Gender (% male): 61 Race/ethnicity (%): white 71; black 22; Asian 0; Hispanic 6 Wound size: 1.74 cm^2 Wound duration >1 year: 100% Comorbid conditions (%): NR	Intervention (n=74): same as above Comparator (n=48): same as above *Antibiotic Use:* NR *Treatment Duration:* 8 weeks *Follow-up Duration:* 6 months *Study Withdrawal (%):* NR for subset of patients *Treatment Compliance:* NR	Allocation concealment: Not applicable to subset Blinding: No Intention to treat analysis (ITT): No Withdrawals/dropouts adequately described: No – number of dropouts in subset not reported
Fumal 2002[79] Belgium Funding Source: NR Therapy Type: Silver Products	Inclusion: at least 2 similar looking chronic leg ulcers; minimal size 16 cm^2; no evidence for clinical infection Exclusion: neurological disorders; arterial occlusion; hypertension; diabetes; intake of antibiotics or any other drug acting on microcirculation or blood coagulation	N=17 patients (34 ulcers) Age (years): 55 NOTE: no other patient characteristics reported	Intervention (n=17 ulcers): 1% silver sulfadiazine cream applied 3x/week Comparator (n=17 ulcers): standard care ALL: saline rinse, hydrocolloid dressing, compression bandage *Antibiotic Use:* NR *Treatment Duration:* 6 weeks *Follow-up Duration:* none *Study Withdrawal (%):* NR *Treatment Compliance:* NR	Allocation concealment: NR Blinding: No Intention to treat analysis (ITT): Yes (no withdrawals reported) Withdrawals/dropouts adequately described: None reported

Study, Year Country Funding Source	Inclusion/Exclusion Criteria	Patient Characteristics Ulcer Type	Intervention Comparator Length of Follow-up	Study Quality
Gentzkow 1996[21] Pilot study for Naughton United States (5 sites) Funding Source: Industry Therapy Type: Biological Skin Equivalent	Inclusion: type 1 or 2 diabetes under reasonable control; ulcers on plantar surface or heel; full-thickness defect >1 cm², wound bed free of necrotic debris/infection and suitable for skin graft (no exposed tendon, bone, or joint; no tunnels or sinus tracts that could not be debrided); adequate circulation (clinical signs and ankle-arm index (AAI) >0.75); ability to complete 12-week trial Exclusion: >1 hospitalization during previous 6 months due to hypoglycemia, hyperglycemia or ketoacidosis; ulcers of nondiabetic origin; use of medications known to interfere with healing (e.g., corticosteroids, immunosuppressives, or cytotoxic agents); pregnancy	N=50 Age (years): 61 Gender (% male): 70 Race/ethnicity (%): NR BMI: NR HbA₁c (%): 8.4 Smoking: NR # Work days missed: NR ABI: ankle-arm index 1.0 Wound location: plantar surface or heel Wound type: diabetic ulcer Wound size: 2.4 cm² Wound grade: NR Wound duration: 55.6 weeks Comorbid conditions (%): NR	Intervention: Dermagraft *Group A* (n=12): weekly (8 pieces & 8 applications) *Group B* (n=14): every 2 wks (8 eight pieces & 4 applications) *Group C* (n=11): every 2 wks (4 pieces & 4 applications) Control *Group D* (n=13): standard wound therapy ALL: sharp debridement; saline-moist gauze; off-loading *Antibiotic Use:* NR *Treatment Duration:* 12 weeks *Follow-up Duration:* mean 14 mos *Study Withdrawal (%):* NR *Treatment Compliance:* NR	Allocation concealment: Adequate Blinding: No Intention to treat analysis (ITT): Yes Withdrawals/dropouts adequately described: No
Hammarlund 1994[72] Sweden Funding Source: NR Therapy Type: Hyperbaric Oxygen (HBOT)	Inclusion: non-diabetic chronic (> 1 year duration) leg ulcers; distal blood pressure at ankle and first digit within normal range (≥100% and ≥70%, respectively, of upper arm blood pressure in mmHg) Exclusion: smoking; concomitant chronic conditions (e.g., diabetes, collagen disease); large vessel disease; ulcers showing tendency to heal (by visual inspection) during 2 months prior to study	N=16 Age (years, median): HBOT 71; control 63 Gender (% male): 50 Race/ethnicity: NR BMI: NR Pre-albumin: NR HbA₁c (%): NR Smoking: 0% (excluded) # Work days missed: NR ABI: NR Wound location: leg Wound type: venous Wound size: 992 mm² Wound grade: NR Wound duration: NR but >1 yr Comorbid conditions (%): History of DM: 0%	Intervention (n=8): HBOT at 2.5 ATA for 90 minutes 5 days/week; multi-place hyperbaric chamber, pressurized for total of 30 sessions over 6 weeks Comparator (n=8): placebo (hyperbaric air) ALL: continued pre-study treatment *Antibiotic Use:* NR *Treatment Duration:* 6 weeks *Follow-up Duration:* 18 weeks (12 from week 6) *Study Withdrawal:* 0 *Treatment Compliance:* 100%	Allocation concealment: Adequate Blinding: Patients, investigators Intention to treat analysis (ITT): Yes (none) Withdrawals/dropouts adequately described: Yes (none)

Advanced Wound Care Therapies for Non-Healing Diabetic, Venous, and Arterial Ulcers: A Systematic Review

Study, Year Country Funding Source	Inclusion/Exclusion Criteria	Patient Characteristics Ulcer Type	Intervention Comparator Length of Follow-up	Study Quality
Hardikar 2005[29] India (8 sites) Funding Source: NR Therapy Type: Platelet-derived Growth Factor	Inclusion: type 1 or 2 diabetes; 18-80 years old; ≥1 full thickness chronic neuropathic ulcer of ≥4 weeks duration; stage 3 or 4 (Wound, Ostomy and Continence Nurses); infection controlled; area 1-40 cm²; adequate perfusion of foot (by ultrasonography, pulse, ABI, ankle or toe pressure) Exclusion: arterial venous ulcers; osteomyelitis or burn ulcers; poor nutritional status (total proteins <6.5 g/dL); uncontrolled hyperglycemia (HbA₁c>12%), persistent infection; life threatening concomitant diseases; foot deformities; chronic renal insufficiency (sCr>3mg/dL); corticosteroid or immunosuppressant use; hypersensitivity to gel components; childbearing age, pregnant or nursing without contraceptive use	N=113 Age (years): 55 Gender (% male): 70 Race/ethnicity (%): native of India: 100 BMI: NR Pre-albumin: NR HbA₁c (%): 7.5 Smoking: NR # Work days missed: NR ABI: 1.06 Wound location: foot Wound type: diabetic Wound size: 12.8 cm² Wound grade: NR Wound duration: 22.6 weeks Comorbid conditions (%): History of DM: 100	Intervention (n=55): 100ug rh-PDGF (0.01%) gel applied daily with volume calculated based on ulcer size Comparator (n=58): placebo gel applied daily ALL: debridement, daily ulcer cleaning and dressing, off-loading *Antibiotic Use:* appropriate use of systemic antibiotics advised *Treatment Duration:* 20 weeks *Follow-up Duration:* NR *Study Withdrawal (%):* 18.6 *Treatment Compliance:* 97.3% (for gel application, dressing changes, and off-loading)	Allocation concealment: Unclear Blinding: Unclear (reported to be double-blind but not specified) Intention to treat analysis (ITT): No Withdrawals/dropouts adequately described: Yes
Harding 2005[60] Multinational – Belgium, United Kingdom, Germany, and Poland (21 sites) Funding Source: Industry Therapy Type: Keratinocytes (LyphoDerm; freeze-dried lysate from cultured allogeneic epidermal keratinocytes)	Inclusion: age 30–85; clinical and documented (refilling time <20 sec or duplex ultrasound in past 12 months) venous insufficiency; no evidence of significant arterial insufficiency (ABI>0.8); ulcer duration >6 wks not healed with std care; size: 1-20 cm² Exclusion: arterial, decubitus, or diabetic ulcer; cellulitis or vasculitis; condition that impairs healing: systemic corticosteroids, immunosuppressive agents, radiation therapy, chemotherapy or surgical treatment/sclero-therapy (past 3 months or planned); bed/wheelchair-bound; clinically significant infected ulcer; consistently bleeding or excessively exudating wound; exposed bone/tendon/fascia; treatment with cell- or growth factor-derived therapies (past month or planned); DVT; other clinical study (past month); allergic to study materials; alcohol or drug abuse (past 5 years); ulcer margin change >3 mm during 4 wk run-in	N=194 (of 200 randomized) Age (years): 67.5 (median) Gender (% male): 39 Race/ethnicity (%): white: 100 BMI: 28.9 (median) Pre-albumin: NR HbA₁c (%): NR Smoking: NR # Work days missed: NR ABI:1.1 (median) Wound location: leg (61% on medial side) Wound type: venous leg ulcers Wound size: 5.2 cm² (median) Wound grade: NR Wound duration: 43 weeks (median) Comorbid conditions (%): History of DM: 6 (12/194)	Intervention (n=95): LyphoDerm 0.9%; 8 applications (wks 0, 1, 2, 3, 4, 6, 8, 10) + standard care (dressing with hydrocolloid and compression therapy) Comparator (n=53): vehicle only + standard care Comparator (n=46): standard care ALL: 4 week run-in period with alginate, hydrocolloid, foam, hydrogel dressings, or petrolatum gauze and compression therapy *Antibiotic Use:* NR *Study Duration:* 28 wks (4 wk run in, 10 wk tx, 14 wk follow up) *Study Withdrawal (%):* 8.2 (16/194) *Treatment Compliance:* 86.6% had no protocol deviation	Allocation concealment: Unclear Blinding: No Intention to treat analysis (ITT): No (excluded 6 patients who weren't treated then one patient from std care group with no baseline data); due to protocol violations, created an "as treated" ITT group (n=193) and a PP group (n=167) Withdrawals/dropouts adequately described: Yes

Advanced Wound Care Therapies for Non-Healing Diabetic, Venous, and Arterial Ulcers: A Systematic Review

Study, Year Country Funding Source	Inclusion/Exclusion Criteria	Patient Characteristics Ulcer Type	Intervention Comparator Length of Follow-up	Study Quality
Harding 2011[66] Europe (43 sites) Funding Source: Industry (reported that sponsor designed study and approved final article; authors had full control over contents of article) Therapy Type: Silver Products	Inclusion: ≥18 years; male or female; ABI ≥0.8; venous leg ulcer (CEAP classification C6); duration <24 months; size 5-40 cm²; ≥3 of the following: pain between dressing changes, perilesional skin erythema, edema, foul odor, or high levels of exudate Exclusion: current antibiotics (week before inclusion; ulcers clinically infected or erysipelas; malignant; recent DVT or venous surgery (past 3 months); progressive neoplastic lesion treated by radiotherapy or chemotherapy; receiving immunosuppressive agents or high dose corticosteroids	N=281 Age (years): 70 Gender (% male): 35 Race/ethnicity: NR BMI: 30 Pre-albumin: NR HbA$_1$c (%): NR Smoking: NR # Work days missed: NR ABI: 1.04 Wound location: 2% foot, 47% ankle, 33% calf, 18% gaiter Wound type: venous Wound size: NR Wound grade: CEAP C6 Wound duration: 0.76 yr Comorbid conditions (%): NR	Intervention (n=145): AQUACEL Ag (4 wks); AQUACEL (4 wks) Comparator (n=136): Urgotul Silver (4 wks); Urgotul (4 wks) ALL: compression; dressing changes per clinical condition & exudate; cleansing; mechanical debridement if needed *Antibiotic Use:* NR *Treatment Duration:* 8 weeks *Follow-up Duration:* none *Study Withdrawal (%):* 8% AQUACEL; 12% Urgotul *Treatment Compliance:* NR	Allocation concealment: Adequate Blinding: Unclear Intention to treat analysis (ITT): Modified (had at least one exposure to treatment) Withdrawals/dropouts adequately described: Yes
Ieran 1990[70] Italy Funding Source: NR Therapy Type: Electromagnetic (EMT)	Inclusion: skin lesions (ulcers due to idiopathic chronic venous insufficiency or post-phlebitic venous insufficiency) present at least for 3 months Exclusion: patients treated with steroids or affected by systemic diseases; concomitant arterial occlusive disease	N=37 (of 44 randomized) Age (years): 66 Gender (% male): 38 Race/ethnicity: NR BMI: NR, Obese 51% Pre-albumin: NR HbA$_1$c (%): NR Smoking: NR # Work days missed: NR ABI: NR Wound location: leg Wound type: venous Wound size: <15 cm² - EMT 54% (mean 4.8), control 46% (5.0); >15 cm² - EMT 36% (mean 34.2), control 64% (39.9) Wound duration: 26 months Comorbid conditions (%): History of DM: 19	Intervention (n=22): EMT stimulator (single pulse of electrical current generating a magnetic field of 2.8 mT at a frequency of 75 Hz, with an impulse width of 1.3 ms for 3-4 hours daily) Comparator (n=22): sham EMT ALL: no elastic compression *Antibiotic Use:* as needed *Treatment Duration:* 90 days or until wound healed *Follow-up Duration:* at least one yr *Study Withdrawal (%):* 16% (n=7) *Treatment Compliance:* Average stimulator use per day (hours) – intervention 3.8, control 3.7	Allocation concealment: Adequate Blinding: Patients, investigators Intention to treat analysis (ITT): No Withdrawals/dropouts adequately described: Yes

Study, Year Country Funding Source	Inclusion/Exclusion Criteria	Patient Characteristics Ulcer Type	Intervention Comparator Length of Follow-up	Study Quality
Jacobs 2008[39] United States Funding Source: NR Therapy Type: Silver Sulfadiazine Cream (SSC)	Inclusion: Wagner grade 1 or 2 ulcerations of the foot; ulcer size 3 cm diameter or less; located on plantar aspect of foot; under care for diabetes mellitus; demonstration of biphasic or triphasic arterial sounds on arterial Doppler; ABI of ≥0.75 Exclusion: HbA$_1$c greater than 10%; non-palpable pulses or history of claudication or rest pain; clinical evidence of local sepsis (absence of malodor, exudates, or erythema extending >1 cm from the ulceration)	N=40 Age (years): NR Gender (% male): NR Race/ethnicity: NR BMI: NR Pre-albumin: NR HbA$_1$c (%): ≤10% for inclusion Smoking: NR # Work days missed: NR ABI: ≥0.75 for inclusion Wound location: plantar Wound type: diabetic ulcer Wound size: 3 cm diameter or less for inclusion Wound grade: Wagner 1 or 2 Wound duration: NR Comorbid conditions (%): History of DM: 100	Intervention (n=20): Bensal HP applied daily Comparator (n=20): SSC applied every 12 hours ALL: debride; off-loading of weight bearing and shoe pressure Antibiotic Use: NR Treatment Duration: 6 weeks Follow-up Duration: none Study Withdrawal (%): 0 Treatment Compliance: NR	Allocation concealment: Unclear Blinding: Yes Intention to treat analysis (ITT): Yes Withdrawals/dropouts adequately described: Yes (none)
Jaiswal 2010[32] India Funding Source: NR Therapy Type: Platelet-derived Growth Factors	Inclusion: type I or type II diabetes and chronic ulcers of at least 4 weeks duration; IAET stage III and IV Exclusion: ankle brachial pressure index (ABI) <0.9	N=50 Age (years): 53 Gender (% male): 84 Race/ethnicity: NR BMI: 22.4 Pre-albumin: NR HbA$_1$c (%): NR Smoking (%): 18 # Work days missed: NR ABI: NR Wound location: lower limb Wound type: diabetic Wound size: 28.2 cm^2 Wound grade: IAET class III – 62%; class IV – 38% Wound duration (median wks): Intervention 5; Control 6 Infection: NR Comorbid conditions (%): History of DM: 100 History of amputation or previous ulcer: 4% History of PVD: 0%	Intervention (n=25): topical rhPDGF gel (PLERMIN) applied once daily Comparator (n=25): topical KY Jelly applied once daily ALL: off-loading in patients with plantar ulcers Antibiotic Use: NR Treatment Duration: 10 weeks Follow-up Duration: NR Study Withdrawal (%): NR Treatment Compliance: NR	Allocation concealment: Adequate Blinding: Unclear Intention to treat analysis (ITT): Yes Withdrawals/dropouts adequately described: Yes

Study, Year Country Funding Source	Inclusion/Exclusion Criteria	Patient Characteristics Ulcer Type	Intervention Comparator Length of Follow-up	Study Quality
Jørgensen 2005[77] Europe and North America (7 countries, 15 sites) Funding Source: Industry Therapy Type: Silver Products	Inclusion: chronic venous or mixed venous/arterial leg ulcer with delayed healing process (area reduction of ≤0.5 cm in past 4 wks); ABI ≥0.65; compression therapy for 4 wks prior to inclusion; ulcer size ≥2 cm²; max of 1.5 cm from edge of 10X10 cm dressing; at least 1 of a) increased exudate (past 4 wks), b) increased ulcer area pain (past 4 wks, per patient), c) discoloration of granulation tissue, d) foul odor (per study personnel) Exclusion: clinical infection; current use of antiseptics/antibiotics (1 wk prior to inclusion & through study); HbA₁c >10%, current systemic corticosteroids >10mg/d or other immunosuppressants from 4 wks prior to inclusion; disease that may interfere with healing	N=129 Age (years): 74 (median) Gender (% male): 36 Race/ethnicity: NR BMI: NR Pre-albumin: NR HbA₁c (%): NR Smoking: NR # Work days missed: NR ABI: 1.0 Wound location: "leg" Wound type: venous or mixed venous/arterial Wound size: 6.4 cm² (median) Wound grade: NR Wound duration: 1.05 years (median) Comorbid conditions (%): NR	Intervention (n=65): sustained release silver foam dressing (Contreet Foam) Comparator (n=64): foam dressing without added silver (Allevyn Hydrocellular) ALL: compression therapy; dressing in place as long as clinically possible (max=7 days) *Antibiotic Use:* Excluded *Treatment Duration:* 4 weeks *Follow-up Duration:* none *Study Withdrawal (%):* 15.5% *Treatment Compliance:* NR	Allocation concealment: Adequate Blinding: No (open study) Intention to treat analysis (ITT): For safety outcomes; per-protocol analysis for performance outcomes Withdrawals/dropouts adequately described: Yes
Jude 2007[40] United Kingdom, France, Germany, Sweden (18 sites) Funding Source: Industry Therapy Type: Silver Products (dressing)	Inclusion: type 1 or 2 diabetes with HbA₁c ≤12%; serum creatinine ≤200 µmol/l; Grade 1 or 2 (Wagner) diabetic foot ulcer of non-ischemic etiology Exclusion: allergic to dressing components; known or suspected malignancy local to the study ulcer; taking systemic antibiotics >7 days prior to enrollment; inadequate arterial perfusion (ABI<0.8, great toe SBP<40 mmHg, or forefoot TcPO₂ <30 mmHg (supine) or <40 mmHg (sitting))	N=134 Age (years): 60 Gender (% male): 74 Race/ethnicity: NR BMI: NR Pre-albumin: NR HbA₁c (%): 8.0 Smoking: NR # Work days missed: NR ABI: 1.8 Wound location: 68% plantar; 32% non-plantar Wound type: 75.5% neuropathic, 24.5% neuroischemic Wound size: 3.7 cm² Wound grade (%): Wagner I 75.5; Wagner II 24.5 Wound duration: 1.3 yrs Comorbid conditions (%): History of DM: 100%	Intervention (n=67): sterile, non-woven sodium carboxymethyl-cellulose primary ionic silver (AQAg, 1.2%) dressing; in place up to 7 days or as indicated Comparator (n=67): sterile, non-woven calcium alginate (CA) dressing (moistened for use on dry wounds, changed daily on infected wounds) ALL: off-load of plantar ulcers *Antibiotic Use:* at clinician's discretion (15.5% at enrollment) *Treatment Duration:* 8 weeks or to healing *Follow-up Duration:* none *Study Withdrawal (%):* 16 *Treatment Compliance:* NR	Allocation concealment: Adequate Blinding: No Intention to treat analysis (ITT): No (final wound evaluation for 65 of 67 in each group) Withdrawals/dropouts adequately described: Yes

127

Advanced Wound Care Therapies for Non-Healing Diabetic, Venous, and Arterial Ulcers: A Systematic Review

Study, Year Country Funding Source	Inclusion/Exclusion Criteria	Patient Characteristics Ulcer Type	Intervention Comparator Length of Follow-up	Study Quality
Karatepe 2011[43] Turkey Funding Source: NR Therapy Type: Negative Pressure Wound Therapy	Inclusion: diabetic foot ulcer Exclusion: none reported	N=67 Age (years): 67.3 Gender (% male): 28 Race/ethnicity: NR BMI: NR Pre-albumin: NR HbA₁c (%): 85% poor control Smoking: NR # Work days missed: NR ABI: 93% > 0.7 Wound location: foot Wound type: diabetic ulcer Wound size: 32.4 cm² Wound grade: NR Wound duration: 9.9 weeks Comorbid conditions (%): History of DM: 100	Intervention (n=30): Negative Pressure Wound Therapy (no details provided) Comparator (n=37): Standard wound care (no details provided) *Antibiotic Use:* NR *Treatment Duration:* NR *Follow-up Duration:* 1 month after healing (mean of 4 months) *Study Withdrawal (%):* 0 *Treatment Compliance:* NR	Allocation concealment: Unclear Blinding: No Intention to treat analysis (ITT): Yes – no withdrawals Withdrawals/dropouts adequately described: Yes – no withdrawals
Kenkre 1996[71] United Kingdom Funding Source: Industry Therapy Type: Electromagnetic (EMT)	Inclusion: venous ulcer with unsatisfactory healing for at least the previous 4 weeks Exclusion: none reported	N=19 Age (years): 71 (Group 1 (59) significantly younger than Group 2 (78) & Comp. (73)) Gender (% male): 26 Race/ethnicity: NR BMI: NR Pre-albumin: NR HbA₁c (%): NR Smoking: NR # Work days missed: NR ABI: NR Wound location: leg Wound type: venous Wound size: EMT 600 Hz: 63 mg (6 to 269) EMT 800 Hz: 81 mg (46 to 197) Control: 119 mg (35 to 526) Wound duration: 626 weeks Comorbid conditions (%): NR	Intervention 1 (n=5): EMT (Elmedistraal) - 600 Hz electric field and 25 mT magnetic field Intervention 2 (n=5): EMT (Elmedistraal) - 600 Hz electric field days 1-5 and 800 Hz days 6-30, and 25 mT magnetic field Comparator (n=9): sham (placebo) *Antibiotic Use:* NR *Treatment Duration:* 30 min week days for a total of 30 days *Follow-up Duration:* 4-week observation period (dressing changes only; final assessment on day 50 *Study Withdrawal (%):* 0	Allocation concealment: Unclear Blinding: Patients, investigators (reported as double-blind) Intention to treat analysis (ITT): Yes (no dropouts) Withdrawals/dropouts adequately described: Yes (no dropouts)

128

Advanced Wound Care Therapies for Non-Healing Diabetic, Venous, and Arterial Ulcers: A Systematic Review

Study, Year Country Funding Source	Inclusion/Exclusion Criteria	Patient Characteristics Ulcer Type	Intervention Comparator Length of Follow-up	Study Quality
Kessler 2003[48] France Funding Source: Foundation Therapy Type: Hyperbaric Oxygen (HBOT)	Inclusion: type 1 and type 2 diabetes; chronic foot ulcers (Wagner grades I, II, and III) Exclusion: gangrenous ulcers, severe arteriopathy (TcPo2<30 mmHg), emphysema, proliferating retinopathy, claustrophobia	N=27 (of 28 randomized) Age (years): 64 Gender (% male): 70 Race/ethnicity: NR BMI: 29.5 Pre-albumin: NR HbA$_1$c (%): 8.8 Smoking: NR # Work days missed: NR ABI: NR Wound location: heel/sole 61%, toe 39% Wound type: diabetic Wound size: 2.6 cm^2 Wound grade: Wagner I–III Wound duration: ≥3 months Comorbid conditions (%): History of CAD/CVD: 22 History of DM: 100	Intervention (n=15): HBOT; 2.5 ATA for two 90-min daily sessions of 100% O$_2$ breathing; multi-place hyperbaric chamber pressurized; 5 days/wk for 2 consecutive wks Comparator (n=13): Wound mgmt ALL: multi-disciplinary wound management program (off-loading, metabolic control, antibiotics) *Antibiotic Use:* 63% *Treatment Duration:* 2 weeks *Follow-up Duration:* 4 weeks *Study Withdrawal (%):* 4% (n=1) *Treatment Compliance:* NR; hospitalized for first 2 weeks	Allocation concealment: Unclear Blinding: Outcome assessors (surface area of the ulcer) Intention to treat analysis (ITT): No, one withdrawal not included in analysis Withdrawals/dropouts adequately described: Yes.
Krishnamoorthy 2003[56] Multinational (6 sites) Funding Source: Industry Therapy Type: Biological Skin Equivalent	Inclusion: full thickness venous leg ulcer without exposure of muscle, tendon or bone; venous reflux in veins of superficial or deep systems; ulcer duration ≥2 months but ≤ 60 months; size of 3-25 cm^3; ABPI ≥ 0.7; < 50% healing from screening visit to day of first intervention (with use of multi-layer compression bandage during 14 day screening period) Exclusion: other causes of ulceration (rheumatoid vasculitis, diabetic foot ulcer); severe leg edema (could not be controlled with compression bandages); soft-tissue infections that would interfere with wound healing; impaired mobility; any underlying medical condition (e.g., PVD, renal disease)	N=53 Age (years): 69 Gender (% male): 42 Race/ethnicity (%): Caucasian: 94; black: 4, Asian: 2 BMI: 30.4 HbA$_1$c (%): NR Smoking: NR # Work days missed: NR ABI: 1.1 Wound location: leg Wound type: venous Wound size (median): 7.0 cm^2 Wound grade: NR Wound duration (median): 47.7 days Infection: NR Comorbid conditions (%): NR	Intervention: compression and Group 1 (n=13): 1 piece of Dermagraft applied weekly during the first 11 weeks (12 applications) Group 2 (n=13): 1 piece of Dermagraft applied at day 0, weeks 1, 4 and 8 (4 applications) Group 3 (n=14): 1 piece of Dermagraft applied at day 0 Comparator (n=13): compression therapy alone (Profore) *Antibiotic Use:* as needed *Treatment Duration:* 11 weeks *Follow-up Duration:* NR *Study Withdrawal (%):* 11.3 *Treatment Compliance:* NR	Allocation concealment: Adequate Blinding: No Intention to treat analysis (ITT): Yes Withdrawals/dropouts adequately described: No

129

Study, Year Country Funding Source	Inclusion/Exclusion Criteria	Patient Characteristics Ulcer Type	Intervention Comparator Length of Follow-up	Study Quality
Landsman 2008[20] United States (4 sites) Funding Source: NR Therapy Type: Collagen Compared with Biological Skin Equivalent	Inclusion: ≥18 years, insulin or non-insulin dependent diabetes; HbA$_1$c 5.5-12%; diabetic ulcer; epidermal ulcers without exposed bone or tendon; viable wound bed with granulated tissue (bleeding following debridement), ulcer size 1-16 cm²; present ≥4 weeks Exclusion: malnourished; allergic to porcine products; hypersensitivity to Dermagraft; severe arterial disease (ABI <0.9); radiation at ulcer site; corticosteroids or immune suppressant use; immunocompromised; non-diabetic ulcer; vasculitis; severe rheumatoid arthritis; severe infection at wound site; osteomyelitis, necrosis, or avascular ulcer bed; hemodialysis; uncontrolled diabetes; active Charcot's neuroarthropathy	N=26 Age (years): 63 Gender (% male): 69 Race/ethnicity: NR BMI: NR Pre-albumin: NR HbA$_1$c (%): NR Smoking: NR # Work days missed: NR ABI: NR Wound location: NR Wound type: diabetic ulcer Wound size: 1.9 cm² Wound grade: NR Wound duration: NR Comorbid conditions (%):NR	Intervention (n=13): extracellular matrix (OASIS); max of 8 applications Comparator (n=13): living skin equivalent (Dermagraft); max of 3 applications with reapplication at 2 and 4 wks if wound closure not achieved ALL: debrided and cleansed; saline moistened gauze left in place for 1 wk; off-loading (boot) *Treatment Duration:* 12 weeks *Follow-up Duration:* 8 weeks *Study Withdrawal (%):* NR *Treatment Compliance:* NR	Allocation concealment: Adequate Blinding: No Intention to treat analysis (ITT): Yes Withdrawals/dropouts adequately described: No
Lindgren 1998[58] Sweden Funding Source: Industry Therapy Type: Biological Skin Equivalent, Cryopreserved	Inclusion: out-patients; venous ulcers over medial part of the distal third of the legs as determined by clinical impression and ABI (cutoff not given) Exclusion: none reported	N=27 Age (years): 76 (median) Gender (% male): 33.3 Race/ethnicity: NR BMI: NR HbA1c (%): NR Smoking: NR # Work days missed: NR ABI: 1.0 Wound type: venous Wound size: 6.3 cm² Wound duration: <2 years: 44.4% >2 years: 55.6% Comorbid conditions (%): NR	Intervention (n=15): keratinocyte allograft + dressing (Mepitel) Comparator (n=12): dressing only ALL: CO2 laser debridement; if infection-free ≥1 wk then pneumatic compression, treatment & elastic compression; inspected on day 3; tx weekly; in bed for 24 hrs; feet elevated when sitting *Antibiotic Use:* as needed *Treatment Duration:* 8 weeks *Follow-up Duration:* 8 weeks *Study Withdrawal (%):* 0% *Treatment Compliance:* NR	Allocation concealment: Unclear Blinding: No Intention to treat analysis (ITT): Unclear Withdrawals/dropouts adequately described: No

Advanced Wound Care Therapies for Non-Healing Diabetic, Venous, and Arterial Ulcers: A Systematic Review

Study, Year Country Funding Source	Inclusion/Exclusion Criteria	Patient Characteristics Ulcer Type	Intervention Comparator Length of Follow-up	Study Quality
Londahl 2010[46] Sweden Funding Source: Foundation Therapy Type: Hyperbaric Oxygen (HBOT)	Inclusion: diabetes; ≥1 full-thickness wound; below ankle; >3 months; previously treated at diabetes foot clinic for at least 2 months; adequate distal perfusion or nonreconstructable peripheral vascular disease Exclusion: contraindications for hyperbaric treatment (severe obstructive pulmonary disease, malignancy, and untreated thyrotoxicosis); current drug or alcohol misuse; vascular surgery in the lower limbs within the last two months; participation in another study; suspected poor compliance	N=94 Age (years): 69 Gender (% male): 81 Race/ethnicity: NR BMI: NR Pre-albumin: NR HbA$_1$c(%): 7.9 Smoking: 25% current # Work days missed: NR ABI: NR Wound location (%): toe 40; plantar forefoot 26; middle 14; malleoli 6; heel 12; dorsal 1 Wound type: diabetic Wound size: 3.0 cm^2 Wound grade (Wagner) (%): Grade II 26; III 56; IV 18 Wound duration, months: 9.5 Comorbid conditions (%): History of CAD/CVD: MI 29%; stroke 16% History of DM: 100% History of amputation: 11% major; 39% minor History of HTN: 75% History of hyperlipidemia: 88%	Intervention (n=49): HBOT; ATA of 2.5; multi-place hyperbaric chamber; compression of air for 5 minutes followed by 85-min daily (session duration 95 min); 5 days/wk; 8 weeks (40 treatment sessions) Comparator (n=45): placebo (hyperbaric air); same schedule ALL: standard treatment at multi-disciplinary diabetes foot clinic (debride, off-load, treatment of infection, revascularization, metabolic control) *Antibiotic Use:* Allowed *Treatment Duration:* 8 weeks *Follow-up Duration:* 1 year *Study Withdrawal (%):* 20 (n=19) *Treatment Compliance:* 57% attended 40 sessions; 80% attended >35 sessions; compliance with standard tx NR	Allocation concealment: Unclear ("sealed envelopes") Blinding: Patients, investigators, outcome assessments_ Intention to treat analysis (ITT): Yes Withdrawals/dropouts adequately described: Yes

Study, Year Country Funding Source	Inclusion/Exclusion Criteria	Patient Characteristics Ulcer Type	Intervention Comparator Length of Follow-up	Study Quality
Marston 2003[23] United States (35 sites) Funding Source: Industry Therapy Type: Biological Skin Equivalent	Inclusion: ≥18 years; type 1 or 2 diabetes; plantar forefoot or heel ulcer present ≥2 weeks; 1.0–20 cm²; full thickness but no exposed muscle, tendon, bone, or joint capsule; no necrotic debris; healthy vascularized tissue present; ABI >0.7; adequate circulation to the foot (palpable pulse) Exclusion: gangrene on affected foot; underlying Charcot deformity; ulcer size changed (+ or -) by >50% during 2 wk screening; severe malnutrition (albumin <2.0); random blood sugar >450 mg/dl; urine ketones present; nearby non-study ulcer; on systemic corticosteroids, immunosuppressive/cytotoxic agents; AIDS or HIV-positive; at-risk for bleeding; cellulitis, osteomyelitis, or other infection	N=245 (ulcer duration >6wks) Age (years): 56 Gender (% male): 74 Race/ethnicity (%): Caucasian 72; Non-Caucasian 28 BMI: NR HbA₁c (%): NR Smoking: NR # Work days missed: NR ABI: NR (>0.7 for inclusion) Wound location: plantar forefoot (87%) or heel (13%) Wound type: diabetic ulcers Wound size: 2.4 cm² Wound duration: 53 wks (41 wks vs. 67 wks, p=NR) Comorbid conditions (%): History of DM 100	Intervention (n=130): Dermagraft; applied weekly up to 8 times over 12 week study Comparator (n=115): standard wound care ALL: sharp debridement + saline-moistened gauze dressings; ambulatory with diabetic footwear *Antibiotic Use:* NR *Treatment Duration:* 12 weeks *Follow-up Duration:* 1 week follow-up to confirm closure *Study Withdrawal (%):* 19 *Treatment Compliance:* NR	Allocation concealment: Unclear Blinding: Yes Intention to treat analysis (ITT): Yes Withdrawals/dropouts adequately described: No
McCallon 2000[44] United States Funding Source: NR Therapy Type: Negative Pressure Wound Therapy	Inclusion: diabetes; age 18-75 years; non-healing foot ulceration present >1 month Exclusion: venous disease; active infection not resolved by initial debridement; coagulopathy	N=10 (pilot study) Age (years): 52.8 Gender (% male): NR Race/ethnicity: NR BMI: NR Pre-albumin: NR HbA₁c (%): NR Smoking: NR # Work days missed: NR ABI: NR Wound location: 9 forefoot, 1 midfoot Wound type: diabetic ulcer Wound size: NR Wound grade: NR Wound duration: NR Comorbid conditions (%): History of DM: 100	Intervention (n=5): continuous pressure (125 mmHg) for 48 hrs; dressing change then intermittent pressure (125 mmHg); dressing change/assessment every 48 hrs Comparator (n=5): saline moistened gauze; changed every 12 hrs; assessed 3 times/wk ALL: initial surgical debridement; bed rest or strict non-wt bearing *Antibiotic Use:* NR *Treatment Duration:* NR *Follow-up Duration:* Followed until delayed primary closure or wound healed by secondary intention *Study Withdrawal (%):* 0 *Treatment Compliance:* NR	Allocation concealment: Inadequate Blinding: No Intention to treat analysis (ITT): Yes – no withdrawals Withdrawals/dropouts adequately described: Yes – no withdrawals

Study, Year Country Funding Source	Inclusion/Exclusion Criteria	Patient Characteristics Ulcer Type	Intervention Comparator Length of Follow-up	Study Quality
Michaels 2009 a,b[67,68] England (2 locations) Funding Source: Government Therapy Type: Silver Products	Inclusion: active ulceration of lower leg, present for more than 6 weeks Exclusion: insulin-controlled diabetes mellitus; pregnancy; sensitivity or specific contraindications to the use of silver; ABI <0.8 in affected leg; maximum ulcer diameter <1 cm; atypical ulcers (e.g., suspicion of malignancy); coexisting skin conditions or vasculitis; receiving oral or parenteral antibiotic treatment	N=213 Age (years): 71 Gender (% male): 46 Race/ethnicity: NR BMI: NR Pre-albumin: NR HbA₁c (%): NR Smoking: 18.3% # Work days missed: NR ABI: NR Wound location: leg Wound type: venous Wound size: 72% <3 cm diam Wound grade: NR Wound duration: 38.5% present for >12 weeks Comorbid conditions (%): History of CAD/CVD: 14% history of MI or cardiac failure, 8% history of stroke or TIA	Intervention (n=107): silver-donating dressings (list of 6 approved for study) Comparator (n=106): non-silver dressings (any non-antimicrobial low-adherence dressing) ALL: multilayer compression bandage (per local practice); dressings changed weekly unless needed; other interventions used if clinically appropriate *Antibiotic Use:* NR *Treatment Duration:* 12 weeks *Follow-up Duration:* to 1 year after entry *Study Withdrawal (%):* 2.3% *Treatment Compliance:* NR	Allocation concealment: Adequate Blinding: No Intention to treat analysis (ITT): No Withdrawals/dropouts adequately described: Yes
Miller 2010[78] Australia (2 sites) Funding Source Foundation, Government Therapy Type: Silver Products	Inclusion: lower leg ulcer; ABI ≥0.6; diameter ≤15 cm; ≥18 years; no topical antiseptic treatment in week before and no antibiotics 48 hrs before recruitment; no systemic steroids; no diagnosis of diabetes or malignancy related to ulcer; not receiving palliative care; no known contraindications to treatment products; ≥ 1 sign of infection or critical colonization (cellulitis, suppuration, lymphangitis, sepsis, bacteremia, changes in granulation tissue, increased or malodorous exudate, new areas of slough or wound breakdown, impaired or delayed wound healing, increased or new pain) Exclusion: none reported	N=266 (of 281 randomized) Age (years): 80 Gender (% male): 41 Race/ethnicity: NR BMI: NR Pre-albumin: NR HbA₁c (%): NR Smoking: NR # Work days missed: NR ABI: NR Wound location: lower leg 97% Wound type: venous (74%), mixed (26.3%) Wound size: 705 mm² Wound grade: NR Wound duration: 54 weeks Comorbid conditions (%): History of DM: 0	Intervention (n=140): Acticoat (silver); clinician chose dressing Comparator (n=141): Iodosorb (iodine); clinician chose dressing ALL: treated until signs of critical colonization and infection absent 1 wk; non-antimicrobial dressing if no signs; required adherence to compression bandaging *Antibiotic Use:* 21% (55/266) *Treatment Duration:* 12 weeks *Follow-up Duration:* none *Study Withdrawal (%):* 5 *Treatment Compliance:* Monitored compression bandage adherence	Allocation concealment: Adequate Blinding: No – open label Intention to treat analysis (ITT): No Withdrawals/dropouts adequately described: Yes

Advanced Wound Care Therapies for Non-Healing Diabetic, Venous, and Arterial Ulcers: A Systematic Review

Study, Year Country Funding Source	Inclusion/Exclusion Criteria	Patient Characteristics Ulcer Type	Intervention Comparator Length of Follow-up	Study Quality
Mostow 2005[53] United States, United Kingdom, Canada (12 Sites) Funding Source: Industry Therapy Type: Biological Dressings	Inclusion: chronic venous insufficiency (clinical presentation, history) and/or positive venous reflux; ≥18 years; ulcer >30 days; 1-49 cm²; between knee and ankle; full thickness and non-healing; visible wound bed with granulation tissue Exclusion: infected, necrotic, or avascular ulcer bed; cellulitis, osteomyelitis, or exposed bone/tendon/fascia; severe RA; uncontrolled CHF or diabetes (HbA₁c >12%); ABI <0.8; history of local radiation; corticosteroids or immune suppressives; known allergy or hypersensitivity to products; sickle cell disease; hemodialysis; malnutrition (albumin <2.5 g/dL); investigational drug or device treatment in last 30 days	N=120 Age (years): 64 Gender (% male): 42 Race/ethnicity (%): white 81; black 16; Asian 1; other 3 BMI: 31.9 HbA₁c (%): NR Smoking: NR # Work days missed: NR ABI: NR, all >0.8 by exclusion Wound type: venous Wound size: 11.1 cm² Wound duration: 1-3 months: 34.2%; 4-6 months: 15.8%; 7-12 months: 10.0%; >12 months: 36.7%; not specified: 3.3% Comorbid conditions (%): NR	Intervention (n=62): OASIS; each week to non-epithelialized portion Comparator (n=58): standard wound care ALL: weekly debride, dressing changes; non-adherent dressing + 4 layer compression bandaging *Antibiotic Use:* NR *Treatment Duration:* 12 weeks; control group offered cross-over to OASIS if not healed; treated for 4 weeks; continued for total of 12 weeks if initial improvement seen *Follow-up Duration:* 6 months; (retained 45% of ITT population) *Study Withdrawal (%):* 20 *Treatment Compliance:* NR	Allocation concealment: Adequate Blinding: No Intention to treat analysis (ITT): Yes Withdrawals/dropouts adequately described: Yes
Naughton 1997[22] United States (20 sites) Funding Source: Industry Therapy Type: Biological Skin Equivalent – Dermagraft	Inclusion: diabetes; neuropathic full-thickness plantar surface foot ulcers of the forefoot or heel; ulcer size >1.0 cm² Exclusion: initial rapid healing in response to standard care during a screening period	N=235 (of 281 randomized) Age (years): NR Gender (% male): NR Race/ethnicity (%): NR BMI: NR HbA₁c (%): NR Smoking: NR # Work days missed: NR ABI: NR Wound location: plantar forefoot or heel Wound type: Diabetic ulcer Wound size: NR Wound duration: NR Comorbid conditions (%): History of DM: 100	Intervention (n=109): Dermagraft; day 0 and weeks 1-7 (8 total) Comparator (n=126): standard wound care ALL: debridement, infection control, saline-moistened gauze dressings, and off-weighting *Antibiotic Use:* NR *Treatment Duration:* 12 weeks (8 week intervention) *Follow-up Duration:* to 32 weeks *Study Withdrawal (%):* 16.4 *Treatment Compliance:* NR	Allocation concealment: Unclear Blinding: "Single-blinded" Intention to treat analysis (ITT): No Withdrawals/dropouts adequately described: No

Study, Year Country Funding Source	Inclusion/Exclusion Criteria	Patient Characteristics Ulcer Type	Intervention Comparator Length of Follow-up	Study Quality
Navratilova 2004[59] Czech Republic Funding Source: Government Therapy Type: Biological Skin Equivalent, cryopreserved versus lyophilized allografts	Inclusion: venous ulcer diagnosed by history, physical examination, and Doppler ultrasonography Exclusion: arterial ulcer; ulcer size <2 cm²; duration <3months; uncompensated diabetes mellitus; pronounced anemia (hg <10.0g/dL); uncompensated heart insufficiency; pronounced hypoproteinemia (albumin <3.5g/dL); ABI <0.8; metastatic malignant tumor; systemic immunosuppressive therapy	N=50 Age (years): 63 Gender (% male): 36 Race/ethnicity: NR BMI: 30.1 HbA$_1$c (%): NR Smoking: NR # Work days missed: NR ABI: NR, >0.8 per exclusion Wound location: leg Wound type: venous ulcer Wound size: 10.7 cm² (cryopreserved 12.4 cm², lyophilized 9.0 cm²) Wound duration: 23.7 months (cryopreserved 21 months, lyophilized 17 months) Comorbid conditions (%): NR	Intervention (n=25): single application of cryopreserved cultured epidermal keratinocytes; nonadherent silicone dressing and gauze bandages; dressings removed after 5 days then changed every 3 days Comparator (n=25): same except allografts of lyophilized cultured epidermal keratinocytes ALL: debride and dressings until clean & granulating wound base achieved; wet saline dressings 1-3 days before graft; hospitalized for graft; bed rest and limb elevation for 48 h after grafting *Antibiotic Use:* systemic; 1 day before allografts if infection *Treatment Duration:* single application *Follow-up Duration:* 3 months *Study Withdrawal (%):* 0% *Treatment Compliance:* NR	Allocation concealment: No Blinding: No Intention to treat analysis (ITT): Yes Withdrawals/dropouts adequately described: None reported

Study, Year Country Funding Source	Inclusion/Exclusion Criteria	Patient Characteristics Ulcer Type	Intervention Comparator Length of Follow-up	Study Quality
Niezgoda 2005[19] United States and Canada (9 Sites) Funding Source: Industry (provided study supplies) Therapy Type: Biological Dressings Compared to Platelet-derived Growth Factors	Inclusion: ≥18 years; type 1 or 2 diabetes; non-healing diabetic ulcer of >30 days; ulcer full thickness with size of 1–49 cm²; visible wound bed with granulation tissue; Grade I, Stage A (UT classification) Exclusion: ulcer of non-diabetic etiology; uncontrolled diabetes (A1C >12%); documented severe arterial disease or low blood supply (TcPO2 <30 mmHg or toe-brachial index <0.70); on corticosteroids or immune suppressives; infected, necrotic, or avascular ulcer bed; cellulitis, osteomyelitis, or exposed bone/tendon/fascia; active Charcot or sickle cell disease; hemodialysis, malnutrition (albumin <2.5 g/dL); known allergy/hypersensitivity to products; treatment with any other investigational drug or device (past 30 days)	N=73 (of 98 randomized) Age (years): 58 Gender (% male): 60 Race/ethnicity %: NR BMI: 32.5 Pre-albumin: NR HbA₁c (%): 8.3 Smoking: NR # Work days missed: NR ABI: NR Wound location: 65% plantar Wound type: diabetic ulcer Wound size: 4.1 cm² Wound duration (%): 1-3 months: 49; 4-6 months: 16; 7-12 months: 15 >12 months: 19 Comorbid conditions (%): History of DM: 100% Type 1 - 49% OASIS, 22% PDGF Type 2 - 51% OASIS, 78% PDGF History of PVD: 0% severe	Intervention (n=37): OASIS; saline and secondary dressing; re-applied weekly as needed Comparator (n=36): PDGF (becaplermin/Regranex); patients applied daily; saline-moistened gauze dressing for 12 hrs then rinsed and covered ALL: off-loading; clean and debride weekly *Antibiotic Use:* NR *Treatment Duration:* 12 weeks; if not healed, crossover tx offered; treated for 4 weeks; continued for total of 12 weeks if initial improvement seen *Follow-up Duration:* 6 months (only 50% of per protocol sample) *Study Withdrawal (%):* 26 *Treatment Compliance:* NR	Allocation concealment: Adequate Blinding: Unclear Intention to treat analysis (ITT): No Withdrawals/dropouts adequately described: Yes
Omar 2004[57] United Kingdom Funding Source: Unclear ("statistical advice and guidance" from industry) Therapy Type: Biological Skin Equivalent, Dermagraft	Inclusion: chronic venous leg ulcers (based on clinical examination, duplex finding of venous dysfunction [all had evidence of superficial reflux, but no deep venous reflux or DVT]; and exclusion of other causes [especially arterial insufficiency, ABPI >0.9]; duration >12 wks; ulcer area 3–25 cm², clean ulcer bed with healthy granulation tissue Exclusion: none reported	N=18 Age (years): 60 Gender (% male): 61 Race/ethnicity: NR BMI: NR HbA₁c (%): NR Smoking: NR # Work days missed: NR ABI: 1.06 Wound type: venous leg ulcer Wound size: 10.7 cm² Wound duration: 119.3 weeks Comorbid conditions (%): NR	Intervention (n=10): Dermagraft at weeks 0, 1, 4 & 8 Comparator (n=8): non-adherent dressing ALL: cleaning, debridement, four-layer compression bandaging *Antibiotic Use:* NR *Treatment Duration:* 12 weeks *Follow-up Duration:* none *Study Withdrawal (%):* NR *Treatment Compliance:* NR	Allocation concealment: Unclear ("computer-generated code based on the order of admittance to the study") Blinding: Yes (ulcer measurement) Intention to treat analysis (ITT): Unclear Withdrawals/dropouts adequately described: None reported

Study, Year Country Funding Source	Inclusion/Exclusion Criteria	Patient Characteristics Ulcer Type	Intervention Comparator Length of Follow-up	Study Quality
Reyzelman 2009[18] United States (11 sites) Funding Source: Industry (compensation to study personnel and consultants involved in data interpretation and writing; therapy provided at no charge) Therapy Type: Collagen	Inclusion: ≥18 years; type 1 or 2 diabetes; diabetic foot ulcer; 1-25 cm²; absence of infection; adequate circulation to affected extremity (TcPO2 >30 mmHg, ABI 0.70–1.2, or biphasic Doppler waveforms in arteries of lower extremity) Exclusion: poor glycemic control (HbA$_1$c >12%); serum Cr >3.0 mg/dl; sensitivity to antibiotics used in preparation of cellular matrix; non revascularable surgical sites; ulcers probing to bone; wound recently treated with biomedical or topical growth factors	N=85 (of 86 randomized) Age (years): 57 Gender (% male): NR Race/ethnicity (%): NR BMI: 33.8 (based on n=83) HbA$_1$c (%): 7.9 Smoking: NR # Work days missed: NR ABI: NR Wound location (%): toe 28; foot 44; heel 17; other 11 Wound type: diabetic ulcer Wound size: 4.3 cm² Wound duration: 23.1 weeks (Note: range=0-139 weeks) Comorbid conditions (%): History of DM: 100; Type 1 – 8.2; Type 2 – 91.8	Intervention (n=47): single application - 4x4 cm human acellular dermal regenerative tissue matrix graft (GRAFTJACKET); sutured or stapled in place; silver-based non-adherent dressing (Silverlon) applied; secondary dressings as determined by investigator Comparator (n=39): standard care (moist-wound therapy with alginates, foams, hydrocolloids or hydrogels at discretion of physician); dressing changes daily or per treating physician ALL: surgical site prep. before tx; off-load (removable cast walker) *Antibiotic Use:* if infection present *Treatment Duration:* 12 weeks *Follow-up Duration:* none *Study Withdrawal (%):* 8% *Treatment Compliance:* NR	Allocation concealment: Unclear Blinding: No Intention to treat analysis (ITT): Yes (included all but one intervention group patient who was removed from participation due to non-compliance) Withdrawals/dropouts adequately described: Yes
Romanelli 2007[75] Italy Funding Source: Industry Therapy Type: Biological Dressing	Inclusion: >18 years; mixed A/V leg ulcer by clinical and instrumental assessment; venous reflux by Doppler flow studies; ABPI >0.6 and <0.8; ulcer duration >6 weeks; 2.5-10 cm²; >50% granulation tissue on wound bed Exclusion: diabetes; current smoker; ABPI <0.6; clinical signs of wound infection; necrotic tissue on wound bed; known allergy to treatment products; unable to follow protocol	N=54 Age (years): 63 Gender (% male): 48 Race/ethnicity (%): NR BMI: NR HbA$_1$c (%): NR (DM excluded) Smoking: 0 (excluded) # Work days missed: NR ABI: 0.6 to 0.8 Wound type: mixed A/V ulcers Wound size: 6 cm² Wound duration: 7.8 weeks Comorbid conditions (%): History of DM: 0 History of PVD: 100	Intervention (n=27): OASIS Comparator (n=27): Hyaloskin ALL: saline + secondary dressing; no compression; observed 2x/wk; dressing change as needed (approx. 1x/wk); all dressings applied in clinic *Antibiotic Use:* NR *Treatment Duration:* 16 weeks *Follow-up Duration:* none *Study Withdrawal (%):* 7.4 (4/54) *Treatment Compliance:* NR	Allocation concealment: Inadequate (every other patient that was selected by clinician for study) Blinding: No Intention to treat analysis (ITT): No Withdrawals/dropouts adequately described: Yes

Advanced Wound Care Therapies for Non-Healing Diabetic, Venous, and Arterial Ulcers: A Systematic Review

Study, Year Country Funding Source	Inclusion/Exclusion Criteria	Patient Characteristics Ulcer Type	Intervention Comparator Length of Follow-up	Study Quality
Romanelli 2010[76] Italy Funding Source: Industry Therapy Type: Biological dressing	Inclusion: venous or mixed A/V leg ulcer; ABI 0.6-0.8; duration >6 months; size >2.5 cm²; 50% granulation tissue on wound bed Exclusion: clinical signs of infection; ABI <0.6; necrotic tissue on wound bed; known allergy to treatment products; unable to follow protocol	N=50 Age (years): NR Gender (% male): 48 Race/ethnicity (%): NR BMI: NR HbA$_1$c (%): NR Smoking: NR # Work days missed: NR ABI: NR but for inclusion 0.6-0.8 Wound location: leg Wound type: venous or mixed A/V ulcer Wound size: 24.4 cm² Wound duration: 7.1 weeks Comorbid conditions (%): NR	Intervention (n=25): OASIS Comparator (n=25): petroleum-impregnated gauze ALL: moistened with saline + secondary nonadherent dressing; assessed weekly for up to 8 wks; patients changed secondary dressing at home *Antibiotic Use:* NR *Treatment Duration:* 8 weeks *Follow-up Duration:* stated monthly follow-up for 6 months (results not reported) *Study Withdrawal (%):* 4% (2/50) *Treatment Compliance:* NR	Allocation concealment: Unclear Blinding: Unclear Intention to treat analysis (ITT): No Withdrawals/dropouts adequately described: Yes
Saad Setta 2011[36] Egypt Funding Sources: NR Therapy Type: Platelet Rich Plasma	Inclusion: age 40-60 yrs; type 1 or 2 diabetes; normal peripheral platelet count (>150,000 mm³) Exclusion: receiving or had received chemo or radiation therapy in past 3 months; screening serum albumin <2.5 ml/dl or hemoglobin <10.5 mg/dl or platelet count <100x10⁹/l; peripheral vascular disease; bacteria count (study ulcer) >10⁵ organisms/gram tissue;, exposed tendons, ligaments or bone	N=24 Age (years): NR Gender (% male): NR Race/ethnicity: NR BMI: NR Pre-albumin: NR HbA$_1$c (%): NR Smoking: 33.3% # Work days missed: NR ABI: NR Wound location: foot Wound type: diabetic Wound size: 9.4 cm² Wound grade: NR Wound duration: ≥12 weeks Infection: NR Comorbid conditions (%): History of HTN: 70	Intervention (n=12): platelet rich plasma applied twice weekly (intervals of 3-4 days) Comparator (n=12): platelet poor plasma (same schedule) ALL: off-loading of ulcer area *Antibiotic Use:* NR *Treatment Duration:* 20 weeks *Follow-up Duration:* none *Study Withdrawal (%):* NR *Treatment Compliance:* NR	Allocation concealment: Unclear Blinding: No Intention to treat analysis (ITT): Unclear Withdrawals/dropouts adequately described: No (not reported)

Study, Year Country Funding Source	Inclusion/Exclusion Criteria	Patient Characteristics Ulcer Type	Intervention Comparator Length of Follow-up	Study Quality
Schuler 1996[69] United States Funding Source: Industry Therapy Type: Intermittent Pneumatic Compression	Inclusion: age >18 years old; ulcers <50 cm^2; ulcers <2 years old Exclusion: ABI <0.9; cancer; massive leg edema due to congestive heart failure; cellulitis; osteomyelitis; sickle cell disease; use of steroids or vasoconstrictive medications; DVT or pulmonary embolism in previous 6 months; vein ligation or injection sclerotherapy in previous year	N=54 Age (years): 57 Gender (% male): 46 Race/ethnicity: NR BMI: 33 Pre-albumin: NR HbA$_1$c (%): NR Smoking (%): 31 # Work days missed: NR ABI: 1.1 Wound location: NR Wound type: venous ulcer Wound size: 9.9 cm^2 Wound grade: NR Wound duration: 306 days Comorbid conditions (%): NR	Intervention (n=28): below-knee gradient compression elastic stocking + external pneumatic compression; applied daily (1 hour in morning + 2 hours in evening) Comparator (n=26): Unna's boot ALL: leg elevation 2X/day *Antibiotic Use:* NR *Treatment Duration:* 6 months *Follow-up Duration:* NR *Study Withdrawal (%):* 13 *Treatment Compliance:* 93% (4 total dropped for non-compliance)	Allocation concealment: Unclear Blinding: No Intention to treat analysis (ITT): No Withdrawals/dropouts adequately described: Yes
Stacey 2000[62] Australia Funding Source: Government, Industry Therapy Type: Platelet Rich Plasma	Inclusion: venous ulceration based on ABI >0.9, venous refilling time < 25 seconds, blood tests negative for other causes of ulceration Exclusion: none reported	N=86 Age (years): 71 Gender (% male): 42 Race/ethnicity: NR BMI: NR Pre-albumin: NR HbA$_1$c (%): NR Smoking: NR # Work days missed: NR ABI: NR Wound location: leg Wound type: venous ulcer Wound size: 4.9 cm^2 Wound grade: NR Wound duration: 12 weeks Comorbid conditions (%): NR	Intervention (n=42): bandage soaked in platelet lysate in phosphate buffered saline (PBS) Comparator (n=44): placebo (PBS) soaked bandage ALL: compression bandaging; dressings/bandages applied twice weekly *Antibiotic Use:* NR *Treatment Duration:* 9 months *Follow-up Duration:* NR *Study Withdrawal (%):* 9 *Treatment Compliance:* NR	Allocation concealment: Adequate Blinding: Unclear Intention to treat analysis (ITT): Unclear Withdrawals/dropouts adequately described: Yes

Advanced Wound Care Therapies for Non-Healing Diabetic, Venous, and Arterial Ulcers: A Systematic Review

Study, Year Country Funding Source	Inclusion/Exclusion Criteria	Patient Characteristics Ulcer Type	Intervention Comparator Length of Follow-up	Study Quality
Steed 1995, 2006[33,34] United States Funding Source: Industry (responsible for conduct of trial and all analyses) Therapy Type: Platelet-derived Growth Factors	Inclusion: ≥19 years; ulcer area 1-100 cm²; chronic (≥8 weeks duration) non-healing; full-thickness; lower extremity ulcer resulting from diabetes; free of infection; adequate arterial blood supply Exclusion: nursing, pregnant, or of childbearing potential; hypersensitivity to study gel; >3 ulcers; ulcers from large-vessel arterial ischemia, venous insufficiency, pressure, or necrobiosis lipoidica diabeticorum; osteomyelitis; malignant or terminal disease; alcohol or substance abuse; thermal, electrical, or radiation burn wounds at site of target ulcer; receiving corticosteroids, immunosuppressive agents, radiation therapy, or chemotherapy	N=118 Age (years): 61 Gender (% male): 75 Race/ethnicity (%): white: 86; other: 14 BMI: NR Pre-albumin: NR HbA₁c (%): NR Smoking: NR # Work days missed: NR ABI: NR Wound location: foot Wound type: diabetic ulcer Wound size: 7.2 cm² Wound grade: NR Wound duration: 78 weeks Infection: NR Infection: Excluded Comorbid conditions (%): NR	Intervention (n=61): platelet-derived growth factor (PDGF-BB 100ug/g gel) applied once/day by patient or patient caregiver Comparator (n=57): placebo gel applied as above ALL: debridement as needed; instructed on off-loading *Antibiotic Use:* NR *Treatment Duration:* 20 weeks *Follow-up Duration:* NR *Study Withdrawal (%):* 27 *Treatment Compliance:* 98% (weight of gel tube, diary of dressing changes)	Allocation concealment: Adequate Blinding: Unclear Intention to treat analysis (ITT): Yes Withdrawals/dropouts adequately described: Yes

Study, Year Country Funding Source	Inclusion/Exclusion Criteria	Patient Characteristics Ulcer Type	Intervention Comparator Length of Follow-up	Study Quality
Vanscheidt 2007[61] Europe (Hungary, Czech Republic, Germany) Funding Source: NR Therapy Type: Keratinocytes (autologous keratinocytes combined with fibrin sealant: BioSeed-S)	Inclusion: age 18-90; chronic venous leg ulcers (>3-month duration); area 2-50 cm² after sharp debridement (±5%); venous insufficiency (by Doppler sonography with reflux in superficial and/or deep veins, venous refilling time <20 seconds; duplex sonography, or phlebography); ulcer located below knee joint excluding ulcers of distal metatarsal area Exclusion: not able to get/apply compression therapy; ABI <0.8; vasculitis, severe rheumatoid arthritis, or other connective tissue diseases; previous surgery on venous system or sclerotherapy, phlebitis, or DVT in past 3 months; significant medical conditions that impair wound healing (e.g., renal and hepatic insufficiency or uncontrolled diabetes); known hypersensitivity to bovine proteins or other constituents of BioSeed-S (if randomized to that group); pregnant or breast-feeding women, or of childbearing age not using contraception during treatment phase	N=225 Age (years): 67 Gender (% male): 37 Race/ethnicity: NR BMI: 28.6 Pre-albumin: NR HbA₁c (%): NR Smoking: 19.1% # Work days missed: NR ABI: NR, but all >0.8 by criteria Wound location: below knee Wound type: venous leg Wound size: 2-10 cm²: 60.4% (136/225) >10 cm²: 38.7% (87/225) Wound grade: NR Wound duration: 3-12 months: 59.1%(133/225) >12 months: 40.9% (92/225) Comorbid conditions (%): NR	Intervention (n=116): *2 wks before Day 0* – skin biopsy to collect and cultivate autologous keratinocytes *Day 0* – debride, disinfect & rinse; applied autologous keratinocytes within fibrin sealant; pressure dressing; compression therapy; repeated up to 3X in first 3 mos; further applications allowed if >2 wks apart; compression therapy maintained throughout 6 months Comparator (n=109): *Day 0* – Same except non-adherent gauze; continuous compression therapy; sharp debridement and paraffin gauze as needed ALL: debrided, routine dressings and compression for 4 weeks prior to Day 0 (not randomized if responsive to std care after 2 wks) *Antibiotic Use:* NR *Treatment Duration:* up to 3 mos *Follow-up Duration:* 6 mos *Study Withdrawal (%):* NR *Treatment Compliance:* NR	Allocation concealment: Unclear Blinding: No Intention to treat analysis (ITT): Yes Withdrawals/dropouts adequately described: No

141

Study, Year Country Funding Source	Inclusion/Exclusion Criteria	Patient Characteristics Ulcer Type	Intervention Comparator Length of Follow-up	Study Quality
Veves 2001[24] United States (24 sites) Funding Source: Industry Therapy Type: Biological Skin Equivalent	Inclusion: type 1 or 2 diabetes; age 18-80 years; HbA₁c 6-12%; full thickness neuropathic ulcers ≥2 weeks in duration (excluded dorsum of foot and calcaneous); ulcer size 1-16 cm²; dorsalis pedis and posterior tibial pulses audible by Doppler Exclusion: clinical infection at ulcer site; significant lower extremity ischemia; active Charcot's disease; ulcer of non-diabetic pathophysiology; significant medical conditions that would impair healing	N=208 (of 277 randomized) Age (years): 57 Gender (% male): 78 Race/ethnicity: white: 69; African American: 16; Hispanic: 13 BMI: 32 HbA₁c (%): 8.6 Smoking: NR Alcohol: NR # Work days missed: NR ABI: >1.0 54%; <0.8 10% Wound Type: neuropathic diabetic foot ulcer Wound size: 2.9 cm² Wound Duration: 11.3 months Comorbid Conditions (%): NR	Intervention (n=112): Graftskin (Apligraf); at baseline then weekly, if needed, for maximum of 4 weeks (max of 5 application) Comparator (n=96): saline moistened gauze ALL: scheduled dressing changes; off-loading Antibiotic Use: NR Treatment Duration: maximum of 4 weeks Follow-up Duration: 12 weeks with safety evaluation to 3 months Study Withdrawal (%): 21 Treatment Compliance: 98%	Allocation concealment: Adequate- Blinding: No Intention to treat analysis (ITT): Modified (excluded 69 patients during 1 week run-in) Withdrawals/dropouts adequately described: Yes
Veves 2002[16] United States (11 sites) Funding Source: Industry Therapy Type: Collagen	Inclusion: ≥18 years of age; diabetic foot ulcer; ≥30 days duration; Wagner grade 1 or 2; area ≥1 cm³; adequate circulation Exclusion: clinical signs of infection; exposed bone; concurrent condition that may interfere with healing; known alcohol or drug abuse; dialysis; corticosteroids; immunosuppressive agents; radiation or chemotherapy; hypersensitivity to dressing components; inability to be fitted with off-loading device; multiple ulcers on same foot	N=276 Age (years): 58.5 Gender (% male): 74 Race/ethnicity (%): white 63, African American 10; Hispanic 16; Native American 12 BMI: NR Pre-albumin: NR HbA₁c (%): 8.6 Smoking: NR # Work days missed: NR ABI: NR Wound location: foot Wound type: diabetic ulcer Wound size: 2.8 cm² Wound grade: NR Wound duration: 3 months (median) Infection: NR Comorbid conditions (%): NR	Intervention (n=138): collagen & oxidized regenerated cellulose dressing (Promogran); application frequency at clinicians' discretion Comparator (n=138): isotonic sodium chloride solution-moistened gauze ALL: surgical debridement at all study visits; dressing changes according to good clinical practice; off-loading Antibiotic Use: NR Treatment Duration: 12 weeks Follow-up Duration: NR Study Withdrawal (%): 32 Treatment Compliance: >90% (both groups; tx, dressing change)	Allocation concealment: Unclear Blinding: No Intention to treat analysis (ITT): Yes Withdrawals/dropouts adequately described: Yes

Advanced Wound Care Therapies for Non-Healing Diabetic, Venous, and Arterial Ulcers: A Systematic Review

Study, Year Country Funding Source	Inclusion/Exclusion Criteria	Patient Characteristics Ulcer Type	Intervention Comparator Length of Follow-up	Study Quality
Vin 2002[52] France (14 sites) Funding Source: Industry Therapy Type: Collagen	Inclusion: venous leg ulcers; free of infection; ≥30 days duration; ABPI ≥0.8; 2 cm-10 cm in any one dimension(if multiple ulcers largest was selected if ≥3 cm away from any other ulcer) Exclusion: unwilling to wear compression bandage continuously; immobile and unable to care for themselves; medical condition that may interfere with healing including carcinoma, vasculitis, connective tissue disease, and immune system disorders; received topical corticosteroids, immunosuppressive agents, radiation therapy, or chemotherapy in 30 days before study entry	N=73 Age (years): 73 Gender (% male): 35 Race/ethnicity: NR BMI: 28 Pre-albumin: NR HbA$_1$c (%): NR Smoking (%): 8 # Work days missed: NR ABI: 1.1 Wound location: leg Wound type: venous ulcer Wound size: 8.2 cm^2 Wound grade: NR Wound duration: 9.2 months Comorbid conditions (%): History of CAD: 11; History of DM: 14; History of HTN: 49	Intervention (n=37): Promogran dressing + Adaptec (petrolatum-impregnated dressing) Comparator (n=36): Adaptec only ALL: compression bandages; dressing changes 2x/wk or more *Antibiotic Use:* NR *Treatment Duration:* to 12 weeks *Follow-up Duration (mean):* Promogran=65.9 days Adaptec=63.8 days *Study Withdrawal (%):* 26 *Treatment Compliance:* NR	Allocation concealment: Unclear Blinding: Partial (investigator assessment validated by 2 clinicians) Intention to treat analysis (ITT): Yes Withdrawals/dropouts adequately described: Yes
Viswanathan 2011[41] India Funding Source: Industry Therapy Type: Silver Products	Inclusion: type 2 diabetes; Wagner Grade I, II, or III ulcer Exclusion: clinical signs of severe infection; exposed bone; unwilling to participate in study	N=38 (of 40 randomized) Age (years): 59 Gender (% male): NR Race/ethnicity: NR Pre-albumin: NR HbA$_1$c (%): 10.7 Smoking: NR # Work days missed: NR ABI: NR Wound location: plantar (66% fore, 24% mid, 11% hind) Wound type: diabetic ulcer Wound size: 4.6 X 3.3 cm Wound grade: 29.0% I, 31.6% II, 39.5% III Wound duration: 14.5 days Comorbid conditions (%): History of DM: 100 History of PAD: 23.7	Intervention (n=20): diabetic wound cream (polyherbal formulation) Comparator (n=20): silver sulphadiazine cream ALL: daily dressing changes (saline wash, cream applied) *Antibiotic Use:* If ulcers showed clinical signs of infection *Treatment Duration:* unclear *Follow-up Duration:* 5 months *Study Withdrawal (%):* 5 *Treatment Compliance:* NR	Allocation concealment: Unclear Blinding: Unclear Intention to treat analysis: No Withdrawals/dropouts adequately described: Yes

143

Study, Year Country Funding Source	Inclusion/Exclusion Criteria	Patient Characteristics Ulcer Type	Intervention Comparator Length of Follow-up	Study Quality
Vuerstaek 2006[80] Netherlands (2 sites) Funding Source: Industry (no influence on data analysis, data interpretation, writing of report, or manuscript submission) Therapy Type: Negative Pressure Wound Therapy	Inclusion: hospitalized with chronic venous, combined venous and arterial, or microangiopathic leg ulcers (>6 months duration); ambulatory; failed conservative local treatment for ≥6 months Exclusion: age >85 years; use of immune suppression; allergy to wound therapies; malignant or vasculitis origin; ABI <0.6	N=60 Age (years): 72 (median) Gender (% male): 23 Race/ethnicity: NR BMI: NR Pre-albumin: NR HbA$_1$c (%): NR Smoking: 26% # Work days missed: NR ABI: 100 (median) Wound location: leg Wound type: venous (43%), combined arterial/venous (13%), arteriolosclerotic (46%) Wound size: 38 cm^2 Wound grade: NR Wound duration: 7.5 months Comorbid conditions (%): History of DM: 17% (type 2) History of HTN: 43% Immobility: 42%	Intervention (n=30; 28 received tx): vacuum-assisted; permanent negative pressure (125 mmHg) until skin graft + 4 days after graft Comparator (n=30; 26 received tx): daily local wound care and compression therapy until skin graft; standard care after graft ALL: initial necrosectomy; full-thickness punch skin graft when 100% granulation tissue on surface and wound secretion minimal; only toilet and basic hygiene mobility during treatment *Antibiotic Use:* 3.5% at baseline *Treatment Duration:* to closure *Follow-up Duration:* 12 months *Study Withdrawal (%):* 10 *Treatment Compliance:* Inpatients	Allocation concealment: Adequate Blinding: No Intention to treat analysis (ITT): Unclear (ITT for adverse events but unclear for other outcomes) Withdrawals/dropouts adequately described: Yes

Study, Year Country Funding Source	Inclusion/Exclusion Criteria	Patient Characteristics Ulcer Type	Intervention Comparator Length of Follow-up	Study Quality
Wainstein 2011[50] Israel Funding Source: NR, device supplied by manufacturer Therapy Type: Ozone-oxygen Therapy	Inclusion: adult (age ≥18 years); type 2 or type 1 diabetes; Wagner classification stage 2 or 3 or post-debridement stage 4 foot ulcer Exclusion: gangrenous foot ulcer; active osteomyelitis; history of collagen diseases; hyperthyroidism; pregnancy or nursing; HbA$_1$c >10.5%; ABI <0.65; hemoglobin <8 g/dL; liver function tests (alanine transaminase, aspartate transaminase, or c-glutamyl transpeptidase) elevated to more than three times the upper normal limit; serum creatinine >2.5 mg/dL or dialysis; known allergy to ozone	N=61 Age (years): 63 Gender (% male): 62 Race/ethnicity: NR BMI: NR Pre-albumin: NR HbA$_1$c (%): 8.6 Smoking: 8% current # Work days missed: NR ABI: 26% 0.65-0.8; 23% 0.8-1.0; 46% >1.0 Wound location: foot Wound type: diabetic Wound size (cm²): ozone 4.9, sham 3.5 Wound grade: Wagner 2-4 Wound duration: 15.8 years Comorbid conditions (%): History of DM: 100%	Intervention (n=31): ozone-oxygen; *Phase I* – tx sessions 4x/wk for 4 wks or granulation in 50% of wound area; max of 1 day between txs (5 day week); gas concentration: 96% oxygen & 4% (80 lg/ mL) ozone; *Phase II* – tx sessions 2x/wk to complete 12 wk tx; gas concentration: 98% oxygen & 2% (40 lg/mL) ozone Comparator (n=30); sham tx; device circulated room air only ALL: debridement; daily wound dressings as needed; tx sessions=26 min *Antibiotic Use:* as needed *Treatment Duration:* 12 weeks *Follow-up Duration:* none *Study Withdrawal (%):* 44 (27/61) *Treatment Compliance:* NR	Allocation concealment: Unclear Blinding: Double (patient and investigator) Intention to treat analysis (ITT): Yes, all randomized included Withdrawals/dropouts adequately described: Yes

Study, Year Country Funding Source	Inclusion/Exclusion Criteria	Patient Characteristics Ulcer Type	Intervention Comparator Length of Follow-up	Study Quality
Wang 2011[45] Taiwan Funding Source: Research Fund through a University Therapy Type: Hyperbaric Oxygen (HBOT)	Inclusion: chronic non-healing foot ulcers of more than 3 months duration Exclusion: cardiac arrhythmia or pacemaker; pregnancy; skeletal immaturity; malignancy	N=77 (of 86 randomized) Age (years): 62 Gender (% male): NR Race/ethnicity: Asian BMI: NR Pre-albumin: NR HbA$_1$c(%): 8.4 Smoking: NR # Work days missed: NR ABI: 0.99 (HBOT 0.91, control 1.07; p=0.06 between groups) Wound location (%): plantar foot 71; dorsal foot 29 Wound type: diabetic Wound size, cm^2 (median): HBOT 7; control 4 (p=0.06) Wound grade (Wagner) (%): NR Wound duration, months (median): HBOT 6; control 6 Comorbid conditions (%): History of DM: 100%	Intervention: HBOT (n=45, 2 with bilateral ulcers); ATA of 2.5; 90 min 5 days/wk for 4 wks (20 sessions); multi-place hyperbaric chamber + standard treatment Comparator: extracorporeal shockwave therapy (dermaPACE device) (n=41, 5 with bilateral ulcers); dosage dependent on ulcer size – min of 500 impulses at E2 (0.23mJ/ mm^2 energy flux density) at 4 shocks/sec; 2 times/ wk for 3 wks (6 sessions) *Antibiotic Use:* per physician *Treatment Duration:* 3–4 weeks depending on therapy; some subjects received 2nd course *Follow-up Duration:* none *Study Withdrawal (%):* 10 (n=9) *Treatment Compliance:* NR	Allocation concealment: Inadequate (odd-even) Blinding: No Intention to treat analysis (ITT): No Withdrawals/dropouts adequately described: Yes
Wieman 1998[31] United States (23 sites) Funding Source: Industry Therapy Type: Platelet-derived Growth Factors	Inclusion: type I or II diabetes; ≥1 full thickness (IAET stage III or IV) wound of lower extremity present for ≥8 weeks; transcutaneous oxygen tension (TcPo$_2$) ≥30 mmHg Exclusion: osteomyelitis affecting target ulcer; post-debridement ulcer size exceeding 100 cm^2; non-diabetic ulcers; cancer; other concomitant diseases; receiving treatment or medication (radiation therapy, corticosteroids, chemotherapy, or immunosuppressive agents); nursing, pregnant, or of childbearing potential not using contraception	N=382 Age (years): 58 Gender (% male): 67 Race/ethnicity: white: 81; black: 12; Asian: 0.3; Hispanic: 6.3; other: 0.3 BMI: NR Pre-albumin: NR HbA$_1$c (%): NR Smoking: NR # Work days missed: NR ABI: NR Wound location: 55% foot dorsum Wound type: diabetic Wound size: 2.7 cm^2 Wound grade: IAET stage III/IV Wound duration: 49 weeks Infection: NR Comorbid conditions (%): NR	Intervention: becaplermin gel# A) 30ug/g (n=132): amount determined weekly at study visits B) 100ug/g (n=123): amount determined weekly at study visits Comparator (n=127): placebo ALL: daily treatment with gel, sharp debridement; moist saline dressings (2x/day), off-loading *Antibiotic Use:* as needed *Treatment Duration:* 20 weeks *Follow-up Duration:* 3 months *Study Withdrawal (%):* 19 *Treatment Compliance:* 97.4% (no details provided) #Regranex 0.01%	Allocation concealment: Unclear Blinding: Unclear (reported to be double-blind but not specified) Intention to treat analysis (ITT): No Withdrawals/dropouts adequately described: Yes

NR=Not Reported; HbA$_1$c=Hemoglobin A$_1$c; DM=Diabetes Mellitus; HTN=Hypertension; CAD/CVD=Coronary Artery Disease/Cardiovascular Disease; PVD=Peripheral Vascular Disease; ITT=Intention to Treat Analysis; BMI=Body Mass Index; PRP=Platelet Rich Plasma; rhPDGF=recombinant human Platelet-derived Growth Factor; IAET=International Association of Enterostomal Therapy; IPC=Intermittent Pneumatic Compression; ABI=Ankle Brachial Index; NPWT=Negative Pressure Wound Therapy; HBOT=Hyperbaric Oxygen Therapy
*The Wagner grade system is a classification based on 6 wound grades (scored 0 to 5) to assess ulcer depth

Table 2. Primary Outcomes

Study, year	Time of assessment (weeks)	Healed ulcers* % (n/N)		Mean time (± SD or SE)** to ulcer healing		Global assessment		Return to daily activities % (n/N)	
		Treatment	Control	Treatment	Control	Treatment	Control	Treatment	Control
DIABETIC ULCERS									
Collagen									
Blume 2011[15] (Formulated Collagen Gel)	12	45 (14/31) (p=ns)	31 (5/16)						
Reyzelman 2009[18] (Graftskin)	12	69.6 (32/46) (p=0.03)	46.2 (18/39)	5.7 ± 3.5 weeks (n=32) (p=ns)	6.8 ± 3.3 weeks (n=18)				
Veves 2002[16] (Promogran)	12	37 (51/138) (p=ns) / Wound duration <6 months: 45 (43/95); (p=0.056); duration >6 months: 19 (8/43) (p=0.83) / Wagner grade 1 or grade 2 – no difference / Ulcer size <10 cm² or ≥10 cm² – no difference	28 (39/138) / Wound duration <6 months: 33 (29/89) / duration >6 months: 20 (10/49)	7.0 ± 0.4 weeks (p<0.0001)	5.8 ± 0.4 weeks				
Donaghue 1998[17] (Fibracol)	8	48 (24/50) (p=ns)	36 (9/25)	6.2 weeks (p=ns)	5.8 weeks				
Biological Dressings									
Niezgoda 2005[19] (OASIS vs PDGF)	12	49 (18/37) (p=0.06)	28 (10/36)	67 days p=0.25	73 days				
Landsman 2008[20] (OASIS vs. BSE [Dermagraft])	12	76.9 (10/13) (p=ns)	84.6 (11/13)	35.7 ± 41.5 days (p=0.73)	40.9 ± 32.3 days				
Biological Skin Equivalents									
Gentzkow 1996[21] (Dermagraft)	12	Group A: 50.0 (6/12) (p=0.03; A versus D) / Group B: 21.4 (3/14) / Group C: 18.2 (2/11)	Group D: 7.7 (1/13)	Group A: 12 weeks / Group B: >12 weeks / Group C: >12 weeks (medians)	Group D: >12 weeks / p=0.056 when comparing groups A and D (medians)				

Study, year	Time of assess-ment (weeks)	Healed ulcers* % (n/N)		Mean time (± SD or SE)** to ulcer healing		Global assessment		Return to daily activities % (n/N)	
		Treatment	Control	Treatment	Control	Treatment	Control	Treatment	Control
Naughton 1997[22] (Dermagraft)	12 (then followed to 32 weeks)	38.5 (42/109) (p=0.14) Received Metabolically active Dermagraft: 48.7 (37/76) (p=0.008)	31.7 (40/126)	13 weeks (median)	28 weeks (median)				
Marston 2003[23] (Dermagraft)	12	30 (39/130) (p=0.049)	18 (21/115)	Reported that treatment group healed faster (p=0.04)					
Veves 2001[24] (Apligraf)	12	56 (63/112) (p=0.004)	38 (36/96)	65 days (median) p=0.003	90 days (median)				
Edmonds 2009[25] (Apligraf)	12	51.5 (17/33) (p=0.049)	26.3 (10/38)	84 days (median)	Not estimated since <50% had full closure				
DiDomenico 2011[26] (Apligraf vs. Theraskin)	12 / 20	41.3 (7/17) (p=ns) / 47.1 (8/17) (p=ns)	66.7 (8/12) / 66.7 (8/12)	6.9 ± 4.1 weeks (n=8) (p=ns)	5.0 ± 3.4 weeks (n=8)				

Platelet-derived Growth Factor

Study, year	Time of assess-ment (weeks)	Healed ulcers* % (n/N)		Mean time (± SD or SE)** to ulcer healing		Global assessment		Return to daily activities % (n/N)	
		Treatment	Control	Treatment	Control				
Aminian 2000[27] (rhPDGF)	8	57 (4/7) Ulcers (p=0.08)	0 (0/5) Ulcers	6.5 +/- 3.7 weeks	No complete healing				
Agrawal 2009[28] (PDGF)	12	64 (9/14) (p<0.001)	21 (3/14)	NR	NR				
Hardikar 2005[29] (rhPDGF)	10 / 20	71(39/55) (p<0.001) / 85 (47/55) (p<0.05β)	31 (18/58) / 53 (31/58)	46 days (p<0.001) / 57 days (p<0.01)	61 days / 96 days				
Bhansali 2009[30] (rhPDGF)	20	100 (13/13) (p=ns)	100 (11/11)	50.1 +/- 23.4 days (p=0.02)	86.1 +/- 30.7 days				
Wieman 1998[31] (rhPDGF – Becaplermin gel)	20	100µg/g: 50 (61/123) (p=0.007) 30µg/g: 36 (48/132) (p=ns vs. placebo gel)	35 (44/127)	100µg/g: 86 days (p=0.01) 30µg/g: NR	127 days				

148

Advanced Wound Care Therapies for Non-Healing Diabetic, Venous, and Arterial Ulcers: A Systematic Review

Study, year	Time of assess-ment (weeks)	Healed ulcers* % (n/N)		Mean time (± SD or SE**) to ulcer healing		Global assessment		Return to daily activities % (n/N)	
		Treatment	Control	Treatment	Control	Treatment	Control	Treatment	Control
Jaiswal 2010[32] (rhPDGF)	10	60 (15/25) (p=ns)	72 (18/25)						
Steed1995 2006[33,34] (rhPDGF)	20	48 (29/61) (p=0.01)	25 (14/57)	30 to 40 days shorter than control group (p=0.01)					
d'Hemecourt 1998[35] (PDGF [Bercaplermin gel] vs. NaCMC or Std care)	20	Gel: 44 (15/34) (p=0.04 vs. std care, p=ns vs. NaCMC)	NaCMC 36 (25/70) Std care: 22 (15/68)	Gel 85 days (p=ns vs. NaCMC or std care)	NaCMC: 98 days Std care: 141 days				
Platelet Rich Plasma									
Saad Setta 2011[36]	20	100 (12/12) (p=ns)	75 (9/12)	11.5 weeks (p<0.005)	17.0 weeks				
Driver 2006[37]	12	ITT: 33 (13/40) (p=ns) PP: 68 (13/19) (p=ns)	ITT: 28 (9/32) PP: 43 (9/21)	PP: 43 days (mean); 45 days (median) (p=ns)	PP: 47 days (mean); 85 days (median)				
Silver Products									
Belcaro 2010[38] (Silver Ointment)	4	39 (13/34) (p<0.05)	16 (5/32)						
Jacobs 2010[39] (Silver Cream (control tx))	6	40 (8/20) (p=ns)	30 (6/20) (Silver)						
Jude 2008[40] (Silver Dressing)	8 or healing	31 (21/67) (p=ns)	22 (15/67)	53 ± 1.8 days (p=ns)	58 ± 1.7 days	(all p=ns except as noted) Healed or Improved: 87.7% Plantar: 81.4% Non-plantar: 100% Baseline antibiotics: 91.7% (p=0.02) None: 86.8% Neuro: 91.2% Neuro-ischemic: 77.0%	70.8% Plantar: 69.6% Non-plantar: 73.7% Baseline antibiotics: 50.0% None: 73.8% Neuro: 71.7% Neuro-ischemic: 68.4%		
Viswanathan 2011[41] (Silver Cream (control tx))	20 (5 months)			43 ± 26.8 days (p=ns)	44 ± 30.7 days (Silver)				

Study, year	Time of assessment (weeks)	Healed ulcers* % (n/N)		Mean time (± SD or SE)** to ulcer healing		Global assessment		Return to daily activities % (n/N)	
		Treatment	Control	Treatment	Control	Treatment	Control	Treatment	Control
Negative Pressure Wound Therapy									
Blume 2008[42]	Ulcer closure or 112 days	43 (73/169) (p=0.007)	29 (48/166)	96 days (median)	Could not be estimated				
Karatepe 2011[43]	Re-epithelization			4 (1.9) weeks (p<0.05)	5 (1.4) weeks				
McCallon 2000[44]	Satisfactory healing	Patients remained in study until satisfactory healing		23 ± 17.4 days (n=5) (p=ns)	43 ± 32.5 days (n=5)				
Hyperbaric Oxygen Therapy									
Wang 2011[45] (vs. extracorporeal shock wave therapy)	4	First course of treatment 25 (10/40) (p=0.008) Second course 6 (1/17) (p=0.01)	First course of treatment 55 (24/44) Second course 50 (7/14)						
Löndahl 2010[46] (vs. sham)	52	52 (25/48) (p=0.03)	29 (12/42)						
Duzgun 2008[47] (vs. standard/ multi-disciplinary wound therapy)	92	66 (33/50) (p<0.001) Wagner 2 100 (6/6) (p<0.001) Wagner 3 68 (13/19) (p<0.001) Wagner 4 56 (14/25) (p<0.001)	0/50 Wagner 2 0/12 Wagner 3 0/18 Wagner 4 0/20						
Kessler 2003[48] (vs. standard/ multi-disciplinary wound therapy)	4	14 (2/14) (p=ns)	0/13						

Advanced Wound Care Therapies for Non-Healing Diabetic, Venous, and Arterial Ulcers: A Systematic Review

Evidence-based Synthesis Program

Study, year	Time of assessment (weeks)	Healed ulcers* % (n/N)		Mean time (± SD or SE)** to ulcer healing		Global assessment		Return to daily activities % (n/N)	
		Treatment	Control	Treatment	Control	Treatment	Control	Treatment	Control
Abidia 2003[49] (vs. sham)	6	62.5 (5/8) (p=0.12)	12.5 (1/8)						
	26	62.5 (5/8) (p=0.31)	25 (2/8)						
	52	62.5 (5/8) (p=0.03)	0 (0/8)						
Ozone-Oxygen Therapy									
Wainstein 2011[50]	24	40.6 (13/32)	reported as 33% n unclear						
VENOUS ULCERS									
Collagen									
Vin 2002[52] (Promogran)	12	ITT: 49 (18/37) (p=ns) PP: 41% (p=ns)	ITT: 33 (12/36) PP: 31%						
Biological Dressings (BD)									
Mostow 2005[53] (OASIS)	12 weeks 6 months	55 (34/62) (p=0.02) 6 months 67 (20/30) (p=ns)	34 (20/58) 6 months 46 (11/24)						
Biological Skin Equivalents									
Falanga 1998[54] Falanga 1999[55] (Apligraf)	6 months	63 (92/146) (p=0.02) Wound duration >1 yr 47 (34/72) (p<0.005)	49 (63/129) 19 (9/48)	61 days (median) (p=0.003) Duration >1 yr 181 days p < 0.005	181 days (median) Could not be determined				
Krishnamoorthy 2003[56] (Dermagraft)	12	Group 1: 38 (5/13) (p=ns) Group 2: 38 (5/13) (p=ns) Group 3: 7 (1/14) (p=ns)	Group 4: 15 (2/13)						

Advanced Wound Care Therapies for Non-Healing Diabetic, Venous, and Arterial Ulcers: A Systematic Review

Study, year	Time of assessment (weeks)	Healed ulcers* % (n/N)		Mean time (± SD or SE)** to ulcer healing		Global assessment		Return to daily activities % (n/N)	
		Treatment	Control	Treatment	Control	Treatment	Control	Treatment	Control
Omar 2004[57] (Dermagraft)	12	50 (5/10) (p=0.15)	12 (1/8)						
Keratinocytes									
Lindgren 1998[58] (Cryopreserved, allogeneic cells)	8	13 (2/15) (p=ns)	17 (2/12)						
Navratilova 2004[59] (Cryopreserved vs. lyophilized)	12	Cryo-preserved 84 (21/25) (p=ns)	Lyophilized 80 (20/25)	Cryo-preserved 32 days (p=ns)	Lyophilized 27 days				
Harding 2005[60] (Lyophilized, allogeneic) NOTE: Control group is combined standard care and standard care + vehicle groups	24	"As treated ITT cohort" 38 (36/95) (p=0.11) "As randomized ITT cohort" 37 (36/98) (p=0.14)	"As treated ITT cohort" 27 (26/98) "As randomized ITT cohort" 27 (26/95)	139.7 ± 5.6 days (p=0.20)	148.5 ± 5.6 days				
Vanscheidt 2007[61] (Autologous, in fibrin sealant)	6 months	38 (44/116) (p=0.01)	22 (24/109)	176 days (median) (p<0.0001)	Median not reached (>201 days)				
Platelet Rich Plasma									
Stacey 2000[62] (PRP)	39	79 (33/42) (p=ns)	77 (34/44)						
Silver									
Belcaro 2010[38] (Silver Ointment)	4	42 (19/44) (p<0.05)	22 (8/38)						
Bishop 1992[63] (Silver Cream (control tx))	4	0/29 Tripeptide (p=0.01 vs. Silver; p=ns vs. placebo)	21 (6/28) (Silver) 3 (1/29) Tripeptide placebo			5.0‡ (Tripeptide) (p<0.0001 vs. other txs)	3.7 (Silver) 5.0 Tripeptide placebo		
Blair 1988[64] (Silver Dressing)	12	63 (19/30) (p=ns)	80 (24/30)						
Dimakakos 2008[65] (Silver Dressing)	9	81 (17/21) (p=0.02)	48 (10/21)	6.1 weeks (p=NR)	6.4 weeks				

Study, year	Time of assessment (weeks)	Healed ulcers* % (n/N)		Mean time (± SD or SE)** to ulcer healing		Global assessment		Return to daily activities % (n/N)	
		Treatment	Control	Treatment	Control	Treatment	Control	Treatment	Control
Harding 2011[66] (2 Silver Dressings)	8 (4 with silver, 4 without)	17 (24/145) (p=0.09) AQUACEL	15 (21/136) Urgotul			67 (97/145)† AQUACEL (p=0.01)	52 (69/136) Urgotul		
Michaels 2009 a,b[67,68] (Silver Dressing)	12 weeks and 1 year	12 weeks 60 (62/104) 1 year 96 (95/99) (both p=ns)	57 (59/104) 96 (90/94)	67 days (median) (p=ns)	58 days (median)				
Intermittent Pneumatic Compression									
Schuler 1996[69]	26	71 (20/28) (p=ns)	60 (15/25)						
Electromagnetic Therapy									
Ieran 1990[70]	12.9 (day 90)	67 (12/18) (p=0.05)	32 (6/19)	71 days	76 days	Excellent# 28 (5/18) Excellent and good# 83 (15/18) (both p=ns)	Excellent# 11 (2/19) Excellent and good# 53 (10/19)	Patient not restricted in activity 44 (8/18) Activity lasted <6 h 39 (7/18) (both p=ns)	Patient not restricted in activity 58 (11/19) Activity lasted <6 h 11 (2/19)
	52	89 (16/18) (p=0.005)	42 (8/19)						
	1 year follow-up from healing	67 (12/18) (p=0.008)	21 (4/19)						
Kenkre 1996[71]	Day 30	0/10 (p=ns)	11 (1/9)			-Groups A and B2 improved ability to walk up flight of stairs following tx -All groups improved in walking a distance of a block of houses -Baseline: "went out for entertainment less often" 58% (11/19); "less sociable to friends and neighbors" 37% (7/19); "went out visiting less frequently" 63% (12/19) -Day 30: 42% (8/19), 16% (3/19), and 37% (7/19), respectively			
	Day 50	All EMT 20 (2/10) EMT Group 1 20 (1/5) EMT Group 2 20 (1/5) (all p=ns)	22 (2/9)						
Hyperbaric Oxygen Therapy									
Hammarlund 1994[72]	18	25 (2/8) (p=ns)	0/8						

153

Advanced Wound Care Therapies for Non-Healing Diabetic, Venous, and Arterial Ulcers: A Systematic Review

| Study, year | Time of assessment (weeks) | Healed ulcers* % (n/N) | | Mean time (± SD or SE)** to ulcer healing | | Global assessment | | Return to daily activities % (n/N) | |
		Treatment	Control	Treatment	Control	Treatment	Control	Treatment	Control
				ARTERIAL ULCERS					
Chang 2000[73] (Biologic Skin Equivalent – Apligraf)	24	4 weeks 32 (7/21) 8 weeks 62 (13/21) 12 weeks 86 (18/21) 24 weeks 100 (21/21) (p<0.01 at all time points)	4 weeks 0/10 8 weeks 0/10 12 weeks 40 (4/10) 24 weeks Reported to be 75% (of 10 patients)	7 weeks (median) (p=0.002)	15 weeks (median)				
				MIXED LOWER EXTREMITY ULCERS					
Brigido 2006[74] (Collagen)	16	86 (12/14) (p=0.01)	29 (4/14)	11.9 weeks	13.5 weeks				
Romanelli 2007[75] (Biological Dressing - OASIS)	16	81 (21/26) (p<0.001)	46 (11/24)						
Romanelli 2010[76] (Biological Dressing)	8	80 (20/25) (p<0.05)	65 (15/23)	5.4 weeks (p=0.02)	8.3 weeks				
Jørgensen 2005[77] (Silver-releasing Dressing)	4	10 (5/52) (p=ns)	9 (5/57)						
Miller 2010[78] (Silver Dressing)	12	64 (85/133) (p=ns)	63 (84/133)	Reported no significant difference in days to heal					
Fumal 2002[79] (Silver Cream)	NR			15 weeks (p=ns)	16 weeks				
Vuerstaek 2006[80] (NPWT)	At discharge (complete healing)	96 (27/28) (p=ns)	96 (25/26)	29 days (median) (p=0.0001)	45 days (median)				
				AMPUTATION ULCERS					
Armstrong 2005[81] (NPWT)	Wound closure or 112 days	56 (43/77) (p=0.04)	39 (33/85)	56 days (median) (p=0.005)	77 days (median)				

SD=Standard deviation; SE=Standard error; tx=Treatment; Neuro=Neuropathic; ITT=Intention to treat population; PP=Per protocol population; NaCMC=sodium carboxymethylcellulose; PDGF=Platelet-derived growth factors; PRP=Platelet rich plasma; BSE=Biological skin equivalent; NPWT=Negative pressure wound therapy

154

Advanced Wound Care Therapies for Non-Healing Diabetic, Venous, and Arterial Ulcers: A Systematic Review

*Complete healing was defined as follows:

Aminian 2000: 100% epithelialization

Brigido 2006: Complete epithelialization without drainage

Landsman 2008: Full epithelialization without drainage or bleeding

Hardikar 2005: Wound closure with full epithelization and no drainage or scab

Schuler 1996: Complete re-epithelialization of the entire wound bed

Vin 2002: 100% reduction in surface area, confirmed by planimetry and the investigator

Blume 2008: Skin closure (100% re-epithelization) without drainage or dressing requirements

Armstrong 2005: 100% re-epithelialization without drainage

Vuerstaek 2006: 2 stage procedure – preparation of wound for skin grafts (granulation tissue covered 100% of surface and secretion minimal) then transplantation of skin grafts with goal of complete healing; data are provided for complete healing

Wang 2011: Not reported

Löndahl 2010: Completely covered by epithelial regeneration and remained so until the next visit in the study. Wagner grade 4 ulcers were considered healed when the gangrene had separated and the ulcer below was completely covered by epithelial regeneration

Duzgun 2008: Total closure of the wound without the need for surgical intervention in the operating room (complete cure with bedside debridement)

Abidia 2003: Complete epithelialization

Kessler 2003: Not reported

Hammarlund 1994: Not reported

Ieran 1990: Completed epithelialization

Belcaro: Complete closure

Jacobs: Data are ulcers reported as "resolved" at end of 6 week study – primary outcome in study was wound size reduction so no definition of healed ulcers

Jude, Miller: 100% re-epithelialization

Viswanathan: Complete epithelialization either by secondary intention or by split skin graft

Bishop: "Total healing"

Blair: Not reported

Harding: "Healed"

Michaels: Complete epithelialization of the ulcer with no scab

Jørgensen: "Closed"

**Some studies reported median time (as noted)

βSeveral covariates were seen as important to the increased healing witnessed in the rhPDGF group: overall baseline ulcer size (p<0.001), use of antibiotics increased healing in the treatment group from 59% to 78% and placebo group from 22.7% to 36% leading to a significant relationship between antibiotic use and the efficacy of treatment drug (p<0.05)

#Rated by three different physicians unaware of the experimental condition

‡Composite score based on erythema, exudation, and granulation (0 to 9+ with lower scores indicating better physical state)

†Composite endpoint: wound volume reduction and final wound assessment of improvement

155

Table 3. Secondary Outcomes – Part A

Study, year (Treatment)	Ulcers infected during treatment % (n/N) Treatment	Ulcers infected during treatment % (n/N) Control	Amputation % (n/N) Treatment	Amputation % (n/N) Control	Revascularization/ surgery % (n/N) Treatment	Revascularization/ surgery % (n/N) Control	Recurrence % (n/N) Treatment	Recurrence % (n/N) Control	Recurrence, mean or median time to (± SD or SE) Treatment	Recurrence, mean or median time to (± SD or SE) Control	Pain/discomfort % (n/N) Treatment	Pain/discomfort % (n/N) Control
DIABETIC ULCERS												
Collagen												
Reyzelman 2009[18] (Graftskin)	NR*	NR*	2 (1/46) (p=ns)	3 (1/39)	2 (1/46) (p=ns)	0/39						
Veves 2002[16] (Promogran)	12 (17/138) (p=ns)	19 (26/138)										
Donaghue 1998[17] (Fibracol)	Reported no difference in number of infections between groups											
Biological Dressings												
Niezgoda 2005[19] (OASIS vs. PDGF)	18 (9/50) (p=ns)	6 (3/48)					25% (2/8 at 6 months) (p=ns)	33% (2/6 at 6 months)			2 events (# pts not reported)	1 event
Biological Skin Equivalents												
Gentzkow 1996[21] (Dermagraft)	Group A: 17 (2/12) Group B: 29 (4/14) Group C: 27 (3/11) (all p=ns)	Group D: 23 (3/13)					Groups A, B, and C: 0 (of 11 healed) (p=ns)	Group D: 0 (of 1 healed)				
Naughton 1997[22] (Dermagraft)	Reported no difference between groups in occurrence of ulcer infections						Reported recurrence in a "comparable minority" in both groups		12 weeks	7 weeks		

Advanced Wound Care Therapies for Non-Healing Diabetic, Venous, and Arterial Ulcers: A Systematic Review

Study, year (Treatment)	Ulcers infected during treatment % (n/N)		Amputation % (n/N)		Revascularization/ surgery % (n/N)		Recurrence % (n/N)		Recurrence, mean or median time to (± SD or SE)		Pain/discomfort % (n/N)	
	Treatment	Control	Treatment	Control	Treatment	Control	Treatment	Control	Treatment	Control	Treatment	Control
Marston 2003[23] (Dermagraft)	Infection 10.4 (17/163) (p=ns) Osteo-myelitis 8.6 (14/163) (p=ns) Cellulitis 7.4 (12/163) Overall 19.0 (31/163) (p=0.007)	Infection 17.9 (27/151) Osteo-myelitis 8.6 (13/151) Cellulitis 9.3 (14/151) Overall 32.5 (49/151)			8 (13/163) had surgical procedure (p=ns)	15 (22/151)						
Veves 2001[24] (Apligraf)	Infection 10.7 (12/112) (p=0.67) Osteo-myelitis 2.7 (3/112) (p=0.04) Cellulitis 8.9 (10/112) (p=ns)	Infection 13.5 (13/96) Osteo-myelitis 10.4 (10/96) Cellulitis 8.3 (8/96)	6.3 (7/112) (p=0.03)	15.6 (15/96)			5.9 (3/112) (p=0.42)	12.9 (4/96)				
Edmonds 2009[25] (Apligraf)	3 (1/33)[β]	0/39	0/33 (p=ns)	2.6 (1/39)			7 (1/15) (p=ns)	10 (1/10)				
Platelet-derived Growth Factor												
Wieman 1998[31] (rhPDGF)	100µg/g: 29 (36/123) 30µg/g: 23 (30/132) (p=ns)	31 (39/127)					NR Reported to be approximately 30% in all treatment groups at 3 month follow-up; number with follow-up data not reported				100µg/g: 6 (7/123) (p=ns) 30µg/g: 6 (8/132) (p=ns)	2 (2/127)
Steed 2006 1995[33,34] (rhPDGF)	Infection 11 (7/61) (p=ns) Cellulitis 5 (3/61) (p=ns) Overall 11.4% (p=ns)	Infection 16 (9/57) Cellulitis 12 (7/57) Overall 26.3%					26% (p=ns)	46%	8.6 weeks	8.5 weeks	7 (4/61) (p=ns)	11 (6/57)

Advanced Wound Care Therapies for Non-Healing Diabetic, Venous, and Arterial Ulcers: A Systematic Review

Evidence-based Synthesis Program

Study, year (Treatment)	Ulcers infected during treatment % (n/N)		Amputation % (n/N)		Revascularization/ surgery % (n/N)		Recurrence % (n/N)		Recurrence, mean or median time to (± SD or SE)		Pain/discomfort % (n/N)	
	Treatment	Control	Treatment	Control	Treatment	Control	Treatment	Control	Treatment	Control	Treatment	Control
d'Hemecourt 1998[35] (rhPDGF – Becaplermin gel versis NaCMC gel or Std Care)	Gel Cellulitis: 3 (1/34) Osteo-myelitis: 9 (3/34) Infection: 21 (7/34) (all p=ns)	NaCMC Cellulitis: 10 (7/70) Osteo-myelitis: 10 (7/70) Infection: 30 (21/70) Std Cellulitis: 15 (10/68) Osteo-myelitis: 13 (9/68) Infection: 28(19/68)									Gel 6 (3/34) (all p=ns)	NaCMC15 (11/70) Std 15 (10/68)
Platelet Rich Plasma												
Driver 2006[37]							PP: 5 (1/13) (p=ns) at 12 weeks	PP: 0				
Silver Products												
Jude 2008[40] (Silver Ointment)	16 (11/67) (p=ns)	12 (8/67)										
Viswanathan 2011[41] Silver Cream (control tx)	5 (1/20) (p=ns)	0/20					47 (9/19) (p=ns)	42 (8/19)				
Negative Pressure Wound Therapy												
Blume 2008[42]	2.4 (4/169) (p=ns)	0.6 (1/166)	4.1 (7/169) (p=0.04)	10.2 (17/166)								
Hyperbaric Oxygen (HBOT)												
Löndahl 2010[46]			Major 6.1 (3/49) (p=ns)	Major 2.2 (1/45)	Open 0% PTA 12.2 (6/49) (p=ns)	Open 0% PTA 8.9 (4/45)						

Study, year (Treatment)	Ulcers infected during treatment % (n/N)		Amputation % (n/N)		Revascularization/ surgery % (n/N)		Recurrence % (n/N)		Recurrence, mean or median time to (± SD or SE)		Pain/discomfort % (n/N)	
	Treatment	Control	Treatment	Control	Treatment	Control	Treatment	Control	Treatment	Control	Treatment	Control
Duzgun 2008[47]			Minor-distal 8.0[b] (4/50) (p<0.01) Minor-proximal 0/50 (p<0.01)	Minor-distal 48.0[c] (24/50) Minor-proximal 34.0† (17/50)	Debride-ment† 0/50 (p=0.003)	Debride-ment† 18.0 (9/50) [Ulcer grade 2=8 Ulcer grade 3=1]						
Abidia 2003[49]	37.5 (3/8) (p=ns)	25 (2/8)	Major 12.5 (1/8) Minor 12.5 (1/8) (both p=ns)	Major 12.5 (1/8)	0/9 (p=ns)	11.1 (1/9) ††						
Ozone-Oxygen Therapy												
Wainstein 2011[50]	"wound infection" 3.1 (1/32)	"infection" 3.4 (1/29)	0/32	3.4 (1/29)								
VENOUS ULCERS												
Collagen												
Vin 2002[52] (Adaptec)	0 (0/37) (p=0.03)	14 (5/36)									19 (7/37) (p=ns)	11 (4/36)
Biological Dressings (BD)												
Mostow 2005[53] (OASIS)	1.6 (1/62) (p=0.11)	8.6 (5/58)					0 (0 of 19 healed ulcers at 6 months) (p=0.03)	30 (3 of 10 healed ulcers at 6 months)				

Advanced Wound Care Therapies for Non-Healing Diabetic, Venous, and Arterial Ulcers: A Systematic Review

Study, year (Treatment)	Ulcers infected during treatment % (n/N)		Amputation % (n/N)		Revascularization/ surgery % (n/N)		Recurrence % (n/N)		Recurrence, mean or median time to (± SD or SE)		Pain/discomfort % (n/N)	
	Treatment	Control	Treatment	Control	Treatment	Control	Treatment	Control	Treatment	Control	Treatment	Control
Biological Skin Equivalents												
Falanga 1998[54] Falanga 1999[55] (Apligraf)	Cellulitis: 8 (12/146) (p=ns) Infection: Reported no difference between groups	Cellulitis: 8 (10/129)					12 (11/92)[a] (p=0.48) Wound duration >1 yr 18 (13/72) (p=ns)	16 (10/63)[a] 22 (12/54)			Reported no difference in pain between treatment groups	
Krishna-moorthy 2003[56] (Dermagraft)	Reported no differences in incidence of infection between groups											
Keratinocytes												
Navratilova 2004[59] (Cryo-preserved vs lyophilized allografts)											Reported pain significantly reduced (p<0.001) during 1st week after application in both groups	
Harding 2005[60] (Lyophilized, allogeneic.) NOTE: Control group is combined standard care and standard care + vehicle group	14 (13/95) (p=ns)	11 (11/99)					22 (8/36) (p=0.78)	19 (5/26)			Tx Period: 4 (4/95) (p=ns) Follow-up Period: 2 (2/89) (p=ns)	2 (2/99) 0/91
Silver Products												
Bishop 1992[63] (Silver Cream (control tx))							No healed ulcers	At 1 yr 17 (1/6) (Silver) 0/1 (Tri-peptide placebo) (p=ns)				

Study, year (Treatment)	Ulcers infected during treatment % (n/N)		Amputation % (n/N)		Revascularization/ surgery % (n/N)		Recurrence % (n/N)		Recurrence, mean or median time to (± SD or SE)		Pain/discomfort % (n/N)	
	Treatment	Control	Treatment	Control	Treatment	Control	Treatment	Control	Treatment	Control	Treatment	Control
Dimakakos 2009[65] (Silver Dressing)											100% pain-free at 8 wks	62% pain-free at 9 wks
Harding 2011[66] (Silver Dressing)	11 (16/145)*** AQUACEL (p=ns)	9 (12/136) Urgotul										
Michaels 2009a,b[67,68] (Silver Dressing)							Of ulcers healed in 1st year 12 (11/95) (p=ns)	14 (13/90)				
Intermittent Pneumatic Compression												
Schuler 1996[69]											VAS score: 2.0 ± 1.4 (p=ns)	VAS score: 3.1 ± 2.3
Electromagnetic Therapy												
Ieran 1990[70]	Day 90 3 ulcers	11 ulcers					Among healed ≤90 days: 2 patients; Among healed >90 days: 2 patients; 25 (4 of 16 healed) (p=ns)	Among healed ≤90 days: 3 patients; Among healed >90 days: 1 patient; 50 (4 of 8 healed)			0.7 cm (from baseline 5.1 cm, based on 11 cm analog scale) (p=ns)	1.4 cm (from baseline 5.3 cm, based on 11 cm analog scale)

Study, year (Treatment)	Ulcers infected during treatment % (n/N)		Amputation % (n/N)		Revascularization/ surgery % (n/N)		Recurrence % (n/N)		Recurrence, mean or median time to (± SD or SE)		Pain/discomfort % (n/N)	
	Treatment	Control	Treatment	Control	Treatment	Control	Treatment	Control	Treatment	Control	Treatment	Control
Kenkre 1996[71]	Day 50 0/10 (p=ns)	Day 50 22.2 (2/9)									Pain in analog scale, mm (range) Day1 600Hz 60 (37-76) Day 30 17 (0-44), (p<0.05 from day 1) Day1 800Hz 62 (29-90) Day 30 36 (0-84), (p<0.05 from day 1)	Pain in analog scale, mm (range) Day 1 47 (0-68) Day 30 41 (0-88)

ARTERIAL ULCERS

Study, year (Treatment)	Treatment	Control	Treatment	Control	Treatment	Control	Treatment	Control	Treatment	Control	Treatment	Control
Chang 2000[73] (Apligraf)	14.3 (3/21) (p=ns)	0 (0/10)					4.8 (1/21) (p=ns)	0 (0/10)				

MIXED LOWER EXTREMITY ULCERS

Study, year (Treatment)	Treatment	Control	Treatment	Control	Treatment	Control	Treatment	Control	Treatment	Control	Treatment	Control
Brigido 2006[74] (Collagen))	21 (3/14) (p=ns)	36 (5/14)[†]										
Romanelli 2007[75] (Biological Dressing - OASIS)											3.7** (p<0.05)	6.2**
Romanelli 2010[76] (Biological Dressing - OASIS)	0/25 (p=ns)	0/25									0/25 (p=ns)	0/25

Advanced Wound Care Therapies for Non-Healing Diabetic, Venous, and Arterial Ulcers: A Systematic Review

Study, year (Treatment)	Ulcers infected during treatment % (n/N)		Amputation % (n/N)		Revascularization/ surgery % (n/N)		Recurrence % (n/N)		Recurrence, mean or median time to (± SD or SE)		Pain/discomfort % (n/N)	
	Treatment	Control	Treatment	Control	Treatment	Control	Treatment	Control	Treatment	Control	Treatment	Control
Jørgensen 2005[77] (Silver-releasing Dressing)											Both groups reported de-creased pain during treatment	
Vuerstack 2006[80] (NPWT)	0 (p=ns)	3 (1/30)					52 (12/23) (p=ns)	42 (10/24)	4th month (median) (p=ns)	2nd month (median)	Pain as AE: 10 (3/30) (p=ns) SF-MPQ[d] Baseline: 9 (4) 8 weeks: 1 (1) PPI[e] Baseline: 2.5 (1) 8 weeks: 0.2 (0.7) (both p<0.05)	3 (1/30) 10 (3) 1 (1) 3.1 (1) 0.4 (0.6)

AMPUTATION ULCERS

Armstrong 2005[81] (NPWT)	17 (13/77) (p=0.04)	6 (5/85)	3 (2/77) (p=0.06)	11 (9/85)								

NR=Not Reported, NPWT=Negative Pressure Wound Therapy; PTA=Percutaneous Transluminal Angioplasty; VAS=Visual Analog Scale for pain (0-100 mm); NaCMC=sodium carboxymethylcellulose; PDGF=Platelet-derived growth factors; PRP=Platelet rich plasma; BSE=Biological skin equivalent; NPWT=Negative pressure wound therapy

[†] No patient required antibiotic treatment or hospital stay. Numbers include infection at the wound site such as periwound erythema or local cellulitis

[*] Any infections were treated and not otherwise reported unless leading to a further adverse event

[**] Pain at end of treatment (VAS with 0=none, 10=severe)

[ß] One patient reported as having multiple infections (osteomyelitis during treatment, and cellulitis during follow-up)

[†] Debridement=operative surgical debridement of the wound was all that was required to achieve closure

[††] Required an "urgent vascular intervention"

[***] Infection and infestation

[a] Measured as recurrence at 12 months in those with complete wound closure at 6 months

[b] HBOT: distal wounds Wagner 3=1; Wagner 4=3

[c] Control: distal wounds Wagner 2=4; Wagner 3=17; Wagner 4=3. Proximal wounds Wagner 4=17

[d] Short Form-McGill Pain Questionnaire (SF-MPQ: 0-45, with 45 reflecting maximum sensory and affective score); mean (SD); significant decrease over time

[e] Present Pain Intensity (PPI: 1-5, mild to excruciating); mean (SD);significant decrease over time and significantly lower in VAC group at baseline and 8 weeks

163

Table 4. Secondary Outcomes – Part B

Study, year (Treatment)	Hospitalization % (n/N)		Required home care % (n/N)		Quality of life Mean/median (±SD/SE)		Other (note) % (n/N)		Other (note) % (n/N)	
	Treatment	Control	Treatment	Control	Treatment	Control	Treatment	Control	Treatment	Control
DIABETIC ULCERS										
Biological Skin Equivalents										
Marston 2003[23] (Dermagraft)							Surgical procedure related to study ulcer: 8 (13/163) (p=0.07)	15 (22/151)		
Negative Pressure Wound Therapy										
Karatepe 2011[43]					Reported positive effect of NPWT on mental (p=0.03) & physical (p=0.004) health (SF=36) compared to standard treatment					
McCallon 2000[44]							Delayed primary closure 80 (4/5) (p=ns)	Delayed primary closure 40 (2/5)		
Hyperbaric Oxygen Therapy										
Löndahl 2010[46]	Leading to study withdrawal 6.1 (3/49) (p=ns)	4.4 (2/45)								
VENOUS ULCERS										
Biological Dressings										
Mostow 2005[53] (OASIS)	Hospitalization resulting in failing to complete study 3 (2/62) (p=ns)	0/58								

Study, year (Treatment)	Hospitalization % (n/N)		Required home care % (n/N)		Quality of life Mean/median (±SD/SE)		Other (note) % (n/N)		Other (note) % (n/N)	
	Treatment	Control	Treatment	Control	Treatment	Control	Treatment	Control	Treatment	Control
Keratinocytes										
Harding 2005[60] (Lyophilized, allogeneic) NOTE: Control group is combined standard care and standard care + vehicle group	2 (2/95) (p=ns)	1 (1/99)								
Platelet Rich Plasma (PRP)										
Stacey 2000[62]			Reported 2 hospitalizations leading to withdrawal but group not reported							
Silver Products										
Michaels 2009a,b[67,68] (Silver Dressing)					EQ-5D 12 weeks 0.73 (n=81) 1 year 0.75 (n=61) SF-6D 12 weeks 0.69 (n=73) 1 year 0.71 (n=55) (all p=ns)	12 weeks 0.70 (n=76) 1 year 0.668 (n=58) 12 weeks 0.70 (n=68) 1 year 0.67 (n=53)				
MIXED LOWER EXTREMITY ULCERS										
Romanelli 2007[75] (OASIS)							Mean time to dressing change 6.4 ±1.4 days	2.4 ±1.6 (p<0.05)	Comfort w/ treatment 2.5 (p<0.01) (0=excellent, 10=critical)	6.7

Advanced Wound Care Therapies for Non-Healing Diabetic, Venous, and Arterial Ulcers: A Systematic Review

Study, year (Treatment)	Hospitalization % (n/N)		Required home care % (n/N)		Quality of life Mean/median (±SD/SE)		Other (note) % (n/N)		Other (note) % (n/N)	
	Treatment	Control	Treatment	Control	Treatment	Control	Treatment	Control	Treatment	Control
Jørgensen, 2005[77] (Silver-releasing Dressing)					EQ-5D 0.79 (p=ns) (1=perfect health, 0=death)	0.79	Odor present 19 (10/52) of ulcers (p=0.03)	39 (22.57)	Dressing changes associated with leakage 19 (10/52) (p=0.002)	49 (28/57)
Vuerstack 2006[80] (NPWT)					EQ-DSI[a] Baseline 40 (13) 8 weeks 76 (17)	Baseline 45 (19) 8 weeks 77 (14)	Wound bed prep time (median): 7 days (p=0.005)	17 days	Skin graft survival: 83% (p=0.01)	70%
AMPUTATION ULCERS										
Armstrong 2005[81] Apelqvist 2008[82] NPWT	Inpatient stay, mean days: 10.6 (p=ns)	9.9					Overall procedures, mean #: 43 (p<0.001)	120	Clinic visits, mean #: 4 (p<0.05)	11

NPWT=Negative pressure wound therapy; EQ-5D=EuroQol 5D; SF-6D=Single index measure generated from SF-36 data; SF-36=Short-Form 36
[a]EuroQol Derived Single Index (EQ-DSI) with higher score reflecting better health status; significant increase over time (both groups)

Advanced Wound Care Therapies for Non-Healing Diabetic, Venous, and Arterial Ulcers: A Systematic Review

Table 5. Secondary Outcomes – Part C

Study, year (Treatment)	Withdrawals due to adverse events % (n/N)		Patients with ≥1 adverse event (%) n/N		All-cause mortality % (n/N)		Allergic reactions to treatment % (n/N)		Treatment specific adverse events % (n/N)		Treatment specific adverse events % (n/N)	
	Treatment	Control	Treatment	Control	Treatment	Control	Treatment	Control	Treatment	Control	Treatment	Control
DIABETIC ULCERS												
Collagen												
Blume 2011[15] (Formulated Collagen Gel)	6 (2/33) (p=ns)	0										
Reyzelman 2009[18] (Graftskin)	6 (3/47) (p=ns)	5 (2/39)	Same as WD due to AE	Same as WD due to AE	0/47 (p=ns)	0/39						
Veves 2002[16] (Promogran)			Non-serious AE: 27 (37/138) Serious AE: 18 (25/138) (both p=ns)	Non-serious AE: 25 (34/138) Serious AE: 25 (35/138)	1.4 (2/138) (p=ns)	4.3 (6/138)						
Donaghue 1998[17] (Fibracol)	Reported that overall 7% (5/75) patients withdrew due to AE; no difference between groups											
Biological Dressings												
Niezgoda 2005[19] (OASIS vs. PDGF)			Reported no difference in proportion of patients with complications or AEs		2 (1/50) (p=ns)	0/48						
Biological Skin Equivalents (BSE)												
Gentzkow 1996[21] (Dermagraft)							Reported no adverse device effects					
Naughton 1997[22] (Dermagraft)			Reported no difference between groups in occurrence of intercurrent events									
Marston 2003[23] (Dermagraft)			67 (87/130) (p=ns)	73 (84/115)								

Advanced Wound Care Therapies for Non-Healing Diabetic, Venous, and Arterial Ulcers: A Systematic Review

Study, year (Treatment)	Withdrawals due to adverse events % (n/N)		Patients with ≥1 adverse event (%) n/N		All-cause mortality % (n/N)		Allergic reactions to treatment % (n/N)		Treatment specific adverse events % (n/N)		Treatment specific adverse events % (n/N)	
	Treatment	Control	Treatment	Control	Treatment	Control	Treatment	Control	Treatment	Control	Treatment	Control
Veves 2001[24] (Apligraf)	5.4 (6/112) (p=ns)	9.4 (9/96)			1/208; treatment group not specified							
Edmonds 2009[25] (Apligraf)	3 (1/33) (p=ns)	10 (4/39)	Serious AE (Tx phase) 12 (4/33) (p=ns)	13 (5/39)	3 (1/33) (p=ns)	0 (0/39)	0 (0/33) (p=ns)	0 (0/39)				
DiDomenico 2011[26] (Apligraf vs. Theraskin)			29 (5/17) (p=ns)	25 (3/12)								
Platelet-derived Growth Factor												
Agrawal 2009[28] (PDGF)							7 (1/14) (p=ns)	0 (0/14)				
Hardikar 2005[29] (rhPDGF)	4 (2/55) (p=ns)	5 (3/58)			0/55 (p=ns)	0/58						
Bhansali 2009[30] (rhPDGF)			Reported no adverse events in either group									
Wieman 1998[31] (rhPDGF – Becaplermin gel)	100µg/g: 11 (13/123) 30µg/g: 13 (17/132) (both p=ns)	10 (13/127)			100µg/g: 1 (1/123) 30µg/g: 2 (3/132) (both p=ns)	2 (3/127)						
Jaiswal 2010[32] (rhPDGF)			Reported no local or systemic side-effects in either group									
Steed 2006 1995[33,34] (rhPDGF)			Overall 51 (31/61) (p=ns) Tx Related 16 (10/61) (p=ns)	Overall 60 (34/57) Tx Related 18 (10/57)	0 (p=ns)	4 (2/57)						

168

Study, year (Treatment)	Withdrawals due to adverse events % (n/N)		Patients with ≥1 adverse event (%) n/N		All-cause mortality % (n/N)		Allergic reactions to treatment % (n/N)		Treatment specific adverse events % (n/N)		Treatment specific adverse events % (n/N)	
	Treatment	Control	Treatment	Control	Treatment	Control	Treatment	Control	Treatment	Control	Treatment	Control
d'Hemecourt 1998[35] (PDGF [Becaplermin gel] versus NaCMC or Std Care)	Gel 15 (5/34) (p=ns vs. both controls)	NaCMC 11 (8/70) Std 24 (16/68)	Gel 65 (22/34) (p=ns vs. both controls)	NaCMC 81 (57/70) Std 71 (48/68)	Gel 3 (1/34) (p=ns vs. both controls)	NaCMC 1 (1/70) Std 3 (2/68)			Wound-related events: Gel 21 (7/34) (p=ns vs. both controls)	NaCMC 27 (19/70) Std 37 (25/68)		
Platelet Rich Plasma												
Driver 2006[37]			Total of 122 events, 60 (49%) in PRP group, 62 (51%) in control group (p=ns)		3 (1/40) (p=ns)	3 (1/32)						
Silver Products												
Belcaro 2010[38] (Silver Ointment)	0/34 (p=ns)	0/32	0/34 (p=ns)	0/32			0/34 (p=ns)	0/32				
Jacobs 2010[39] (Silver Cream control tx)	0/20 (p=ns)	0/20	0/20 (p=ns)	0/20			0/20 (p=ns)	0/20				
Jude 2007[40] (Silver Dressing)	12 (8/67) (p=ns)	19 (13/67)	37 (25/67) (p=ns)	39 (26/67)	1.5 (1/67) (p=ns)	1.5 (1/67)			Study-related events 16 (11/67) (p=ns)	13 (9/67)		
Viswanathan 2011[41] (Silver Cream control tx)	5 (1/20) (p=ns)	0/20	0/19 (Per-protocol)	0/19	0/20 (p=ns)	5 (1/20)						
Negative Pressure Wound Therapy												
Blume 2008[42]	11.2 (19/169) (p=ns)	9.0 (15/166)			1.8 (3/169) (p=ns)	1.8 (3/166)						
McCallon 2000[44]	0/5 (p=ns)	0/5			0/5 (p=ns)	0/5						

169

Study, year (Treatment)	Withdrawals due to adverse events % (n/N)		Patients with ≥1 adverse event (%) n/N		All-cause mortality % (n/N)		Allergic reactions to treatment % (n/N)		Treatment specific adverse events % (n/N)		Treatment specific adverse events % (n/N)	
	Treatment	Control	Treatment	Control	Treatment	Control	Treatment	Control	Treatment	Control	Treatment	Control
Hyperbaric Oxygen Therapy												
Löndahl 2010[46]	2.0 (1/49) (p=ns)	6.7 (3/45)			2.0 (1/49) (p=ns)	6.7 (3/45)	Oxygen toxicity 0/49 (p=ns)	0/45	Baro-traumatic otitis 2.0 (1/49)‡ (p=ns)	0/45‡	Dizziness 2.0 (1/49) Worsen cataract 2.0 (1/49)	Minor head injury 2.2 (1/45)
Duzgun 2008[47]	0/50 (p=ns)	0/50										
Kessler 2003[48]	6.7 (1/15) (p=ns)	0/13	6.7 (1/15) (p=ns)	0/13	0/15 (p=ns)	0/13			Baro-traumatic otitis 6.7 (1/15) (p=ns)	0/13		
Abidia 2003[49]	0/9 (p=ns)	11.1 (1/9)*	0/9 (p=ns)	11.1 (1/9)*	0/9 (p=ns)	0/9						
VENOUS ULCERS												
Collagen (COL)												
Vin 2002[52] (Promogran)	14 (5/37) (p=ns)	14 (5/36)					14 (5/37) (p=ns)	14 (5/36)				
Biological Dressings (BD)												
Mostow 2005[53] (OASIS)	9.6 (6/62) (p=ns)	10.3 (6/58)	Reported no difference in proportions of patients with AEs between groups (8 events in OASIS group, 15 in control)		1.6 (1/62) (p=ns)	0/58	3 events in 62 patients	3 events in 58 patients				
Biological Skin Equivalents												
Falanga 1998[54] Falanga 1999[55] (Apligraf)	2.1 (3/146) (p=ns)	5.4 (7/129)			3.4 (5/146) (p=ns)	3.1 (4/129)						

Study, year (Treatment)	Withdrawals due to adverse events % (n/N)		Patients with ≥1 adverse event (%) n/N		All-cause mortality % (n/N)		Allergic reactions to treatment % (n/N)		Treatment specific adverse events % (n/N)		Treatment specific adverse events % (n/N)	
	Treatment	Control	Treatment	Control	Treatment	Control	Treatment	Control	Treatment	Control	Treatment	Control
Krishnamoorthy 2003[56] (Dermagraft)	Group 1: 0/13 Group 2: 1/13 Group 3: Unclear† (all p=ns)	Group 4: 0/13	Group 1: 18 AE's, 1 serious Group 2: 15 AE's, 1 serious Group 3: 15 AE's, 4 serious	Group 4: 17 AE's, 0 serious	No deaths							
Keratinocytes												
Harding 2005[60] (Lyophilized, allogeneic) NOTE: Control group is combined standard care and standard care + vehicle group			Local AE: Tx phase 22 (21/95) Follow-up 8 (7/89) General AE: Tx phase 25 (24/95) Follow-up 16 (14/89) (all p=ns)	23 (23/99) 5.5 (5/91) 23 (23/99) 14 (13/91)	1 (1/95) (p=ns)	0/99	Reported no differences between treatment groups in "sensations such as burning, stinging, pain, or itching"					
Vanscheidt 2007[61] (Autologous, in fibrin sealant)			33 (38/116) (63 events) (p=ns for patients) Serious AEs: 10 (12/116) (12 events)	25 (27/109) (51 events) 10 (11/109) (14 events)	0.9 (1/116) (p=ns)^	0.9 (1/109)						
Platelet Rich Plasma												
Stacey 2000[62]	5 patients withdrew from study w/ allergy to paste bandage and 1 w/ trauma on leg from bandages; not detailed by group											

Advanced Wound Care Therapies for Non-Healing Diabetic, Venous, and Arterial Ulcers: A Systematic Review

Study, year (Treatment)	Withdrawals due to adverse events % (n/N)		Patients with ≥1 adverse event (%) n/N		All-cause mortality % (n/N)		Allergic reactions to treatment % (n/N)		Treatment specific adverse events % (n/N)		Treatment specific adverse events % (n/N)	
	Treatment	Control	Treatment	Control	Treatment	Control	Treatment	Control	Treatment	Control	Treatment	Control
Silver Products												
Belcaro 2010[38] (Silver Ointment)	0/44 (p=ns)	0/38	0/44	0/38 (p=ns)			0/44 (p=ns)	0/38				
Bishop 1992[63] (Silver Cream - control tx)							Reported no statistical differences among treatment groups					
Blair 1988[64] (Silver Dressing)							13 (4/30) (p=ns)	0/30	Deterioration due to cellulitis 7 (2/30) (p=ns)	3 (1/30)		
Dimakakos 2009[65] (Silver Dressing)									0 (0/21) due to tx	0 (0/21) due to tx		
Harding 2011[66] (Silver Dressing)	6 (9/145) AQUACEL (p=ns)	9 (12/136) Urgotul	Any AE 50 (72/145) Related AE 23 (33/145) (both p=ns)	42 (57/126) 18 (24/136)	0/145 (p=ns)	1.4 (2/136)						
Michaels 2009ab[67,68] (Silver Dressing)	1 (1/107) (p=ns)	0/106			12 week tx 0/107 (p=ns) 1st year 4 (4/107) (p=ns)	0/106 4 (4/106)						
Intermittent Pneumatic Compression												
Schuler 1996[69]	4 (1/28) (p=ns)	7.7 (2/26)					0 (0/28) (p=ns)	3.8 (1/26)				
Electromagnetic Therapy												
Ieran 1990[70]	9.1 (2/22)# (p=ns)	0/22			0/22 (p=ns)	0/22						

172

Study, year (Treatment)	Withdrawals due to adverse events % (n/N)		Patients with ≥1 adverse event (%) n/N		All-cause mortality % (n/N)		Allergic reactions to treatment % (n/N)		Treatment specific adverse events % (n/N)		Treatment specific adverse events % (n/N)	
	Treatment	Control	Treatment	Control	Treatment	Control	Treatment	Control	Treatment	Control	Treatment	Control
Kenkre 1996[71]	0/10 (p=ns)	0/9	68 (13/19) Results not reported by treatment arm		0	NR	Moderate/ severe headache 20 (2/10) Sense of heat, tingling, and "needles and pins" in limbs 30 (3/10)	0/9 33 (3/9)				
ARTERIAL ULCERS												
Chang 2000[73] (Biologic Skin Equivalent - Apligraf)	0/21 (p=ns)	0/10	14.3 (3/21) (p=ns)	0/10	4.8 (1/21) (p=ns) (after ulcer had healed)	0/10						
MIXED LOWER EXTREMITY ULCERS												
Brigido 2006[74] (Collagen)			AEs were comparable between treatment arms									
Romanelli 2007[75] (Biological Dressing – OASIS)	0/27 (p=ns)	0/27	0/27 (p=ns)	0/27	0/27 (p=ns)	0/27						
Romanelli 2010[76] (Biological Dressing – OASIS)	0/25 (p=ns)	0/25	0/25 (p=ns)	0/25	0/25 (p=ns)	0/25						
Jørgensen 2005[77] (Silver-releasing Dressing)			Device-related AEs 6 (4/65) (p=ns)	5 (3/64)					↑ ulcer size 14 (9/65) (p=ns)	25 (16/64)		
Miller 2010[78] (Silver Dressing)			8 (13/140) (p=ns)									
Vuerstack 2006[80] (NPWT)			40% (p=ns)	23%	13 (4/30) (p=ns)	7 (2/30)						

173

Study, year (Treatment)	Withdrawals due to adverse events % (n/N)		Patients with ≥1 adverse event (%) n/N		All-cause mortality % (n/N)		Allergic reactions to treatment % (n/N)		Treatment specific adverse events % (n/N)		Treatment specific adverse events % (n/N)	
	Treatment	Control	Treatment	Control	Treatment	Control	Treatment	Control	Treatment	Control	Treatment	Control
AMPUTATION ULCERS												
Armstrong 2005[81] (NPWT)			52 (40/77) (p=ns)	54 (46/85)								

AE=Adverse event; PP=Per protocol population; NaCMC=sodium carboxymethylcellulose; PDGF=Platelet-derived growth factors; PRP=Platelet rich plasma; BSE=Biological skin equivalent; NPWT=Negative pressure wound therapy

‡2 patients in each group required myringotomy with tube placement due to pain caused by the inability to equilibrate air pressure through the eustachion tube

#allergic reaction to drugs, diagnosed as having rheumatoid arthritis

†3 withdrawals reported in text; 2 withdrawals reported in Figure 1 in article; Table 1 in article includes >1 serious adverse event only in Group 3

^1 additional death in screening phase; treatment group not reported

APPENDIX E. COMMON METHODOLOGICAL ERRORS AND RECOMMENDATIONS FOR FUTURE CLINICAL TRIALS OF WOUND HEALING

1. Common Methodological Errors in Studies of Wound Care

Source:

European Wound Management Association
> Gottrup F, Apelqvist J, Price P. Outcomes in controlled and comparative studies on non-healing wounds: recommendations to improve the quality of evidence in wound management. *J Wound Care.* 2010;19:239-68.

- Lack of validation of subjective assessments
- Lack of description of objective or subjective measures
- Lack of comparable baselines for patient groups
- Lack of blinding for the evaluation of primary outcomes
- Incorrect randomization methods
- Poor definition of primary and secondary objectives
- Number of patients not based on *a priori* sample size calculation
- Randomization method poorly/not described
- Time to wound healing not a primary objective
- Intention-to-treat analysis not used
- Heterogeneous study population
- Number of and reason for dropouts not stated
- No specification of adjuvant treatments
- Small sample size combined with multiple outcome measures
- Reporting of multiple outcomes over multiple time points (increased chance of type 1 error)
- Poor overall study reporting

2. Recommendations for Clinical Trials of Wound Healing

Sources:

Center for Medical Technology Policy
> Center for Medical Technology Policy. Effectiveness Guidance Document: Methodological Recommendations for Comparative Effectiveness Research on the Treatment of Chronic Wounds. Version 2.0, October 1, 2012. Available at: http://www. cmtpnet.org/effectiveness-guidance-documents/negative-pressure-wound-therapy-egd/. Accessed October 2012.

European Wound Management Association
> Gottrup F, Apelqvist J, Price P. Outcomes in controlled and comparative studies on non-healing wounds: recommendations to improve the quality of evidence in wound management. J Wound Care. 2010;19:239-68.

Panel on Wound Care Evidence-Based Research

Serena T, Bates-Jensen B, Carter MJ, et al. Consensus principles for wound care research obtained using a Delphi process. Wound Repair Regen. 2012;20:284-93.

US Food and Drug Administration

FDA. Guidance for Industry: Chronic Cutaneous Ulcer and Burn Wounds-Developing Products for Treatment. 2006. Available at: http://www.fda.gov/downloads/Drugs/GuidanceComplianceRegulatoryInformation/Guidances/UCM071324.pdf. Accessed September 2012.

1. "Chronic" needs to be defined or replaced with "non-healing."
2. Studies should be multi-center to include a range of settings.
3. Studies should focus on one wound type with stratification by risk factors for not healing.
4. Exclusion criteria should be minimal to increase generalizability; rationale for inclusion and exclusion criteria should match the goals of the study.
5. Randomization is critical; baseline wound characteristics have a major effect on outcomes. Non-randomized trials should be considered only when there are barriers to conducting randomized trials that can be identified and explained.
6. Interventions should be clearly described and consistent across all patients.
7. Simultaneous and/or sequential interventions should be evaluated when appropriate.
8. Standard care should be clearly defined and consistent across study sites or balanced using stratification of study sites for multi-site studies; large cohort studies with each wound type should establish outcomes achieved with standard care.
9. Protocols for pain management and treatment of comorbid conditions should be standardized in all study arms.
10. Comparator arms in studies of dressings, medications, etc. should be a "vehicle control arm" with the same components except for the active agent; if the effect of the "vehicle" is not known, there should also be a standard care group only.
11. Blinding of subjects and investigators should be employed if feasible; blinded assessment by a third-party evaluator should be considered if blinding of investigators and patients isn't possible.
12. Outcome assessment tools should be pre-specified and protocols standardized across patients and across study sites for multi-site studies.
13. The patient population should be appropriate for the treatment and type of wound to be studied.
14. A substantial proportion of patients should be drawn from clinical settings where wound care is delivered.
15. Chronic ulcers might heal because patients become more compliant with standard therapy when enrolled in a trial; studies should include a run-in period of standard care (1-2 weeks) with entry criterion based on change in ulcer size during the run-in phase to exclude those healing because of compliance.
16. Endpoints should be chosen based on the purpose of the intervention; important outcomes include:
    a. incidence of complete closure (defined as skin re-epithelialization without drainage or dressing requirements confirmed at two consecutive study visits 2 weeks apart); closure should be confirmed by an independent source; trial should include at least

3 months follow-up following closure to distinguish actual healing from transient wound coverage; partial healing should not be a primary endpoint except partial healing to facilitate surgical wound closure; if purpose of intervention is something other than healing, endpoints should be pre-defined and validated scoring systems used,

b. accelerated wound closure (decreased time to healing); monitoring intervals should be sufficiently short to detect meaningful difference in time to closure between treatment groups; ideally all patients would be followed until healing is achieved,

c. quality of healing (e.g., scarring, contour and feel of healed skin, normalization of skin markings or pigmentation),

d. quality of wound care (e.g., prevention or cure of infection, reduced pain and/or decreased blood loss with debridement, pain), and

e. activities of daily living, quality of life, limb salvage, dressing performance.

17. Potential sources of bias include:

a. selection bias – allocation concealment is important,

b. performance bias – clearly define standard care; blind outcome assessment; include independent assessment of outcomes,

c. attrition bias – document reasons for drop-out; plan for drop-outs, including withdrawals due to wound deterioration,

d. detection bias – define outcomes; follow-up to detect recurrence, and

e. publication bias – trials may not be published or available in indexed journals.

18. National or formal wound registries should be developed.